Curbside Consultation
in Cornea and External Disease

49 Clinical Questions

Price
Vision Group

Please accept this book in thanks for the opportunity of working with you to serve your patients. Your trust in Price Vision Group is greatly valued by everyone at our office and serves as a reminder that our efforts to maintain the highest quality standards have not gone unnoticed. We hope you find this book useful in your practice.

Francis W. Price Jr., MD

Kathy Kelley, OD   *Faye Peters, OD*

Curbside Consultation in Ophthalmology
Series

SERIES EDITOR, DAVID F. CHANG, MD

Curbside Consultation
in Cornea and External Disease

49 Clinical Questions

EDITOR

Francis W. Price, Jr, MD
Price Vision Group
Indianapolis, Indiana

ASSOCIATE EDITORS

Marianne O. Price, PhD
Cornea Research Foundation of America
Indianapolis, IN

Erik Letko, MD
Price Vision Group
Indianapolis, Indiana

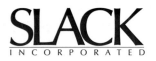

ISBN: 978-1-55642-931-6

Published by: SLACK Incorporated
                 6900 Grove Road
                 Thorofare, NJ 08086 USA
                 Telephone: 856-848-1000
                 Fax: 856-853-5991
                 www.slackbooks.com

Contact SLACK Incorporated for more information about other books in this field or about the availability of our books from distributors outside the United States.

Library of Congress Cataloging-in-Publication Data

Curbside consultation in cornea and external disease : 49 clinical questions / editor, Francis W. Price Jr ; associate editors, Marianne Price, Erik Letko.
       p. ; cm. -- (Curbside consultation in ophthalmology series)
    Includes bibliographical references and index.
    ISBN 978-1-55642-931-6 (alk. paper)
    1. Cornea--Diseases. I. Price, Francis W., 1951- II. Price, Marianne O., 1952- III. Letko, Erik. IV. Series: Curbside consultation in ophthalmology series.
       [DNLM: 1. Corneal Diseases--complications. 2. Contact Lenses--adverse effects. 3. Cornea--injuries. WW 220 C977 2010]
    RE336.C867 2010
    617.7'19--dc22
                                        2010000815

Last digit is print number: 10 9 8 7 6 5 4 3 2 1

Dedication

We dedicate this to ophthalmologists everywhere, who in the normal course of caring for their patients, encounter patients for whom a curbside consult with a cornea specialist would be helpful.

Contents

Acknowledgments

Wendy Mickler is the wind beneath our wings. We enormously appreciate her dedication, perseverance, organizational skills, way with words, and sense of humor in bringing this project to fruition.

About the Editor

Francis W. Price, Jr., MD, founder and medical director of Price Vision Group in Indianapolis, IN, is an internationally recognized ophthalmic surgeon and recipient of the Senior Achievement Award from the American Academy of Ophthalmology. He has authored over 100 peer-reviewed publications and has been principal investigator on over 80 clinical studies of ophthalmic devices, medications, and surgical techniques. He is also an inventor and holds several patents for ophthalmic devices. Dr. Price is a graduate of Indiana University Medical School and completed a fellowship in cornea and external disease at Tulane University. He has been active in developing and teaching endothelial keratoplasty techniques to hundreds of surgeons from around the world.

About the Associate Editors

Marianne Price, PhD is executive director of the Cornea Research Foundation of America in Indianapolis, IN. She holds a PhD in Medical and Molecular Genetics from Indiana University School of Medicine. A respected scientist and author, Dr. Price has made presentations to vision care audiences around the world. She is a member of the American Academy of Ophthalmology and serves on the Board of Prevent Blindness Indiana, the Indiana University Kelley School of Business—Women MBA's Alumni Advisory Board, and the Scientific Programs and Research Committees of the Eye Bank Association of America. She and Dr. Francis Price are recipients of Melvin Jones Fellow Awards from the Lions International Foundation and Vision Awards from the Corneal Dystrophy Foundation.

Erik Letko, MD dedicates his career to the improvement of treatment and surgical techniques for a spectrum of corneal conditions. He graduated from Charles University 1st School of Medicine in Prague, Czech Republic, where he also completed his ophthalmology residency and cornea fellowship. He received extensive training as a fellow in Cornea, External Eye Diseases, and Ocular Immunology at the Massachusetts Eye and Ear Infirmary, Harvard Medical School. He completed a second residency in ophthalmology at Casey Eye Institute in Portland, OR. Dr. Letko participated in over 30 clinical studies and authored or co-authored over 25 peer reviewed articles and 10 book chapters. He serves as a reviewer for ophthalmology journals and lectures in the United States and abroad.

Contributing Authors

Natalie A. Afshari, MD, FACS (Question 14)
Associate Professor, Ophthalmology
Director, Cornea and Refractive Surgery
    Fellowship
Duke University Eye Center
Durham, NC

Anthony J. Aldave, MD (Question 3)
Associate Professor, Ophthalmology
Director, Cornea Service
Director, Cornea and Refractive Surgery
    Fellowship
The Jules Stein Eye Institute
Los Angeles, CA

Penny Asbell, MD, FACS, MBA (Question 32)
Editor in Chief, *Mount Sinai Journal of
    Medicine*
Professor, Ophthalmology
Director, Cornea and Refractive Services
Department of Ophthalmology
Mount Sinai School of Medicine
New York, NY

Dimitri T. Azar, MD (Question 5)
B.A. Field Chair, Ophthalmologic Research
Professor and Head
Department of Ophthalmology and Visual
    Sciences
Illinois Eye and Ear Infirmary
University of Illinois at Chicago
Chicago, IL

Neal P. Barney, MD (Question 10)
Associate Professor
Department of Ophthalmology and Visual
    Sciences
University of Wisconsin School of Medicine
    and Public Health
Madison, WI

Michael W. Belin, MD (Question 34)
Professor, Ophthalmology & Visual Science
University of Arizona Health Sciences
Southern Arizona Veterans Administration
    Health Care System
Tucson, AZ

Richard E. Braunstein, MD (Question 21)
Director, Anterior Segment and Refractive
    Surgery
Miranda Wong Tang Associate Professor,
    Clinical Ophthalmology
Columbia University
Harkness Eye Institute
New York, NY

Daniel Brocks, MD (Question 32)
Mount Sinai Hospital
Department of Ophthalmology
New York, NY

JoAnn C. Chang, MD (Question 9)
Clinical Instructor
Department of Ophthalmology and Visual
    Sciences
John A. Moran Eye Center
University of Utah
Salt Lake City, UT

David S. Chu, MD (Question 46)
Associate Professor, Ophthalmology
Division of Cornea and Refractive Surgery
Institute of Ophthalmology and Visual
    Science
New Jersey Medical School–UMDNJ
Newark, NJ

John W. Cowden, MD (Question 27)
Chairman and Roy E. Mason Distinguished
    Professor, Ophthalmology
University of Missouri
Department of Ophthalmology
Columbia, MO

Reza Dana, MD, MSc, MPH (Question 24)
Claes H. Dohlman Professor, Ophthalmology
Vice Chairman and Associate Chief,
    Ophthalmology (Academic Programs)
Director, Cornea & Refractive Surgery
    Services
Massachusetts Eye & Ear Infirmary
Senior Scientist and W Clement Stone
    Scholar
Schepens Eye Research Institute
Boston, MA

Muriel Doors, MD (Question 47)
Department of Ophthalmology
University Hospital Maastricht
Maastricht, The Netherlands

James P. Dunn, MD (Question 20)
Wilmer Eye Institute
Division of Ocular Immunology
Johns Hopkins School of Medicine
Baltimore, MD

Brad H. Feldman, MD (Question 14)
Attending Surgeon, Cornea Service
Wills Eye Institute
Philadelphia, PA

Martin Filipec, MD, PhD (Question 27)
Professor, Ophthalmology
Lexum European Eye Clinic
Charles University
Prague, Czech Republic
Advance Visioncare
London, United Kingdom

*C. Stephen Foster, MD, FACR, FACS (Question
    17)*
Clinical Professor, Ophthalmology
Harvard Medical School
Boston, MA
Founder and President, Ocular Immunology
    and Uveitis Foundation
Massachusetts Eye Research and Surgery
    Institution
Cambridge, MA

*Frederick (Rick) W. Fraunfelder, MD (Question
    23)*
Associate Professor, Ophthalmology
Director of Cornea/Refractive Surgery
Casey Eye Institute
Oregon Health and Science University
Portland, OR

Prashant Garg, MD (Question 27)
Faculty, Cornea and Anterior Segment
    Services
Medical Director
Ramayamma International Eye Bank
L. V. Prasad Eye Institute
Hyderabad, India

Jeffrey P. Gilbard, MD (Question 15)

Kenneth Mark Goins, MD (Question 41)
Professor, Clinical Ophthalmology
Medical Director, Iowa Lions Eye Bank
University of Iowa Hospitals and Clinics
Iowa City, IA

Mark S. Gorovoy, MD (Question 1)
Gorovoy MD Eye Specialists
Fort Myers, FL

Jose L. Güell, MD (Question 44)
Associate Professor, Ophthalmology
Universitat Autonoma de Barcelona
Director, Cornea and Refractive Surgery
    Unit
Instituto de Microcirugia Ocular
Barcelona, Spain

Sadeer B. Hannush, MD (Question 2)
Attending Surgeon, Cornea Service, Wills
    Eye Institute
Medical Director, Lions Eye Bank of Delaware
    Valley
Scientific Program Chair, The Cornea
    Society
Assistant Professor, Ophthalmology
Jefferson Medical College
Philadelphia, PA

Bennie H. Jeng, MD (Question 43)
Associate Professor, Ophthalmology
Co-Director, Cornea Service
University of California
Chief, Department of Ophthalmology
San Francisco General Hospital
San Francisco, CA

Albert S. Jun, MD, PhD (Question 16)
Associate Professor, Ophthalmology
Cornea and Anterior Segment Service
Wilmer Eye Institute
Johns Hopkins Medical Institutions
Baltimore, MD

Stephen C. Kaufman, MD, PhD (Question 36)
Lyon Professor, Ophthalmology
Director, Cornea and Refractive Surgery
Department of Ophthalmology
University of Minnesota
Minneapolis, MN

Tanya Khan, BA (Question 31)
Duke University School of Medicine
Durham, NC

Terry Kim, MD (Question 31)
Professor, Ophthalmology
Duke University School of Medicine
Director, Fellowship Programs
Associate Director, Cornea and Refractive
    Surgery
Duke University Eye Center
Durham, NC

Thomas Kohnen, MD (Question 8)
Professor, Ophthalmology
Department of Ophthalmology
Goethe University
Frankfurt am Main, Germany

Aarup A. Kubal, MD (Question 20)
Wilmer Eye Institute
Division of Ocular Immunology
Johns Hopkins School of Medicine
Baltimore, MD

Marian Macsai, MD (Question 35)
Professor, Ophthalmology
University of Chicago Pritzker School of
    Medicine
Chief, Division of Ophthalmology
NorthShore University Healthsystem
Glenview, IL

Francis S. Mah, MD (Question 28)
Associate Professor, Ophthalmology and
    Pathology
University of Pittsburgh School of Medicine
Department of Ophthalmology
Department of Pathology
UPMC Eye Center
Pittsburgh, PA

Mark J. Mannis, MD, FACS (Question 40)
Professor and Chair
Department of Ophthalmology & Vision
    Science
University of California
Davis Health System Eye Center
Sacramento, CA

Thomas F. Mauger, MD (Question 38)
Chair, Department of Ophthalmology
Ohio State University
Columbus, OH

*Jod S. Mehta, BSc, MBBS, MRCOphth,
    FRCOphth, FRCS(Ed) (Question 39)*
Consultant, Corneal and External Eye
    Disease and Refractive Service
Singapore National Eye Centre
Clinician Scientist
Assistant Director, Clinical Trials
Head, Tissue Engineering and Stem Cells
    Group
Singapore Eye Research Institute
Adjunct Associate Professor, Duke-NUS
    Graduate Medical School Singapore
Adjunct Associate Professor, Department of
    Ophthalmology
Yong Loo Lin School of Medicine
National University of Singapore
Singapore

Merce Morral, MD (Question 44)
Instituto de Microcirugia Ocular
Institut Clínic d'Oftalmologia, Hospital
  Clinic i Provincial de Barcelona
Barcelona, Spain

Majid Moshirfar, MD, FACS (Question 9)
Professor, Ophthalmology
Director, Cornea & Refractive Surgery
  Division
Department of Ophthalmology and Visual
  Sciences
John A. Moran Eye Center
University of Utah
Salt Lake City, UT

John D. Ng, MD, MS, FACS (Question 22)
Associate Professor
Departments of Ophthalmology and
  Otolaryngology/Head & Neck Surgery
Casey Eye Institute
Oregon Health and Sciences University
Devers Eye Institute
Portland, OR

Rudy M. M. A. Nuijts, MD, PhD (Question 47)
Associate Professor, Ophthalmology
Department of Ophthalmology
University Hospital Maastricht
Maastricht, The Netherlands

Michael A. Page, MD (Question 23)
Oregon Health & Science University
Casey Eye Institute
Portland, OR

Carlindo Da Reitz Pereira, MD (Question 33)
Price Vision Group
Indianapolis, IN

Henry Daniel Perry, MD (Question 25)
Senior Founding Partner, Ophthalmic
  Consultants of Long Island
Clinical Associate Professor, Ophthalmology
State University of New York at Stonybrook
Rockville Centre, NY

Stephen C. Pflugfelder, MD (Question 11)
Professor and Director, Ocular Surface
  Center
James and Margaret Elkins Chair
Department of Ophthalmology
Baylor College of Medicine
Houston, TX

Roberto Pineda, MD (Question 42)
Director, Refractive Surgery
Massachusetts Eye and Ear Infirmary
Assistant Professor, Ophthalmology
Harvard Medical School
Boston, MA

Yaron S. Rabinowitz, MD (Question 37)
Director, Cornea Genetic Eye Institute
Cedars-Sinai Medical Center
Clinical Professor of Ophthalmology
UCLA School of Medicine
Los Angeles, CA

Michael B. Raizman, MD (Question 18)
Ophthalmic Consultants of Boston
Director, Cornea and Cataract Service
New England Eye Center
Associate Professor of Ophthalmology
Tufts University School of Medicine
Boston, MA

J. Bradley Randleman, MD (Question 7)
Associate Professor, Ophthalmology
Emory Eye Center & Emory Vision
Department of Ophthalmology
Emory University
Atlanta, GA

Virender S. Sangwan, MS (Question 12)
Head, Cornea & Anterior Segment
Ocular Immunology & Uveitis Service
Associate Director, L. V. Prasad Eye Institute
Kallam Anji Reddy Campus
L. V. Prasad Marg, Banjara Hills
Hyderabad, India

Hosam Sheha, MD, PhD (Question 45)
Ocular Surface Center
Ocular Surface Research and Education
    Foundation
Miami, FL

Mohamed Abou Shousha, MD (Question 6)
Department of Corneal and External
    Diseases
Bascom Palmer Eye Institute
University of Miami
Miami, FL

Sana S. Siddique, MD (Question 17)
Research Fellow
Massachusetts Eye Research and Surgery
    Institution
Ocular Immunology and Uveitis
    Foundation
Cambridge, MA

Roger F. Steinert, MD (Question 49)
Chair, Department of Ophthalmology
Director, Gavin Herbert Eye Institute
Irving H. Leopold Professor, Ophthalmology
Professor, Biomedical Engineering
University of California, Irvine
Irvine, CA

Donald Tan, FRCSG, FRCSE, FRCOphth,
    FAMS (Question 39)
Director, Singapore National Eye Centre
Chairman, Singapore Eye Research Institute
Professor, Ophthalmology
Yong Loo Lin School of Medicine
National University of Singapore
Singapore

Joseph Tauber, MD (Question 48)
Clinical Professor, Ophthalmology
Kansas University School of Medicine
Department of Ophthalmology
Tauber Eye Center
Kansas City, MO

Mark A. Terry, MD (Question 4)
Director, Corneal Services
Devers Eye Institute
Scientific Director
Lions Eye Bank of Oregon Vision Research
    Laboratory
Professor, Clinical Ophthalmology
Oregon Health Sciences University
Portland, OR

Kristina Thomas, MD (Question 5)
Cornea Fellow
Department of Ophthalmology and Visual
    Sciences
Illinois Eye and Ear Infirmary
University of Illinois at Chicago
Chicago, IL

Prathima R. Thumma, MD (Question 21)
Cornea Fellow
Columbia University, Harkness Eye Institute
New York, NY

William Trattler, MD (Question 13)
Director of Cornea
Center for Excellence in Eye Care
Miami, FL

Scheffer C. G. Tseng, MD, PhD (Question 45)
Ocular Surface Center
Ocular Surface Research and Education
    Foundation
Miami, FL

Elmer Y. Tu, MD (Question 29)
Director, Cornea and External Disease
    Service
Associate Professor, Clinical Ophthalmology
University of Illinois Eye and Ear Infirmary
Department of Ophthalmology and Visual
    Sciences
University of Illinois at Chicago
Chicago, IL

David D. Verdier, MD (Question 19)
Clinical Professor
Department of Surgery, Ophthalmology
  Division
Michigan State University College of Human
  Medicine
Grand Rapids, MI

Nienke Visser, MD (Question 47)
Department of Ophthalmology
University Hospital Maastricht
Maastricht, The Netherlands

Carroll A. Webers, MD, PhD (Question 47)
Department of Ophthalmology
University Hospital Maastricht
Maastricht, The Netherlands

Jayne S. Weiss, MD (Question 26)
Professor, Ophthalmology and Pathology
Kresge Eye Institute
Wayne State University School of Med-icine
Detroit, MI

Sonia H. Yoo, MD (Question 6)
Professor, Ophthalmology
Bascom Palmer Eye Institute
University of Miami, Miller School of
  Medicine
Miami, FL

Preface

David Chang asked us to come up with a series of questions that general ophthalmologists and residents are likely to encounter in the area of cornea. Practical and concise answers were generously provided by top corneal specialists from around the world—just the type of answers one needs in a busy practice. The international flavor and range of expertise represented in this book is best illustrated by Question 27, in which 3 corneal specialists from different regions of the world each explain their approach to working up and treating a patient who presents with a corneal ulcer.

SECTION I

CORNEAL DEGENERATION AND DYSTROPHY

QUESTION

I Have a Patient With Fuchs' Endothelial Dystrophy. Is There Anything New to Improve Her Vision?

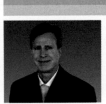

Mark S. Gorovoy, MD

Fuchs' endothelial corneal dystrophy (FECD), defined by the presence of dark spots (guttae) on corneal endothelium (Figure 1-1), is the leading indication for corneal transplant in the Western world. This hereditary condition is rarely symptomatic before the sixth decade of life when gradual reduction in visual acuity sets in (Figure 1-2). First guttae and then corneal edema due to endothelial cell insufficiency contribute to reduction of visual acuity. The quality of vision also becomes affected by halos and glare from bright light or while driving at night. Diurnal fluctuation of visual acuity, worse in the morning, is pathognomonic for this condition. In later stages, epithelial edema and progressive stromal fibrosis may develop, resulting in further decrease of vision. At that point, patients may also experience eye irritation and foreign body sensations from an irregular ocular surface and ruptured epithelial bullae.

Diagnosis

Early diagnosis of FECD is important because this condition may, even in the beginning stages, increase the risk for corneal decompensation with intraocular surgery or corneal procedures such as laser in situ keratomileusis (LASIK). The diagnosis is relatively easy to make once guttae can be visualized bilaterally on slit-lamp examination. Ancillary testing, including specular or confocal microscopy and pachymetry, is typically not necessary for the purpose of diagnosis but becomes helpful when monitoring progression of the disease. In contrast, confocal or specular microscopy in early stages of

3

Figure 1-1. Confluent guttae in a patient with Fuchs's corneal endothelial dystrophy.

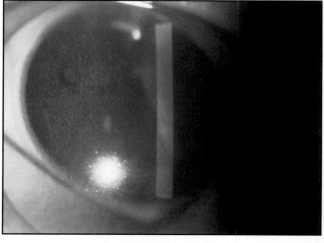

Figure 1-2. Focal corneal edema in a patient with Fuchs's corneal endothelial dystrophy.

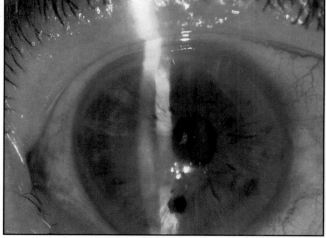

FECD might play a crucial role in diagnosis, particularly during a preoperative evaluation for intraocular or corneal surgery in cases where the degree of suspicion is high and slit-lamp exam is inconclusive.

Treatment

There is essentially no medical treatment for FECD. Hypertonic saline solution has been used to reduce corneal edema, but its efficacy is limited and temporary at best. The treatment is typically indicated when the patient becomes symptomatic. Corneal transplantation offers a definitive solution for a symptomatic patient. Penetrating keratoplasty was the standard of treatment for corneal decompensation secondary to FECD. Due to a long vision rehabilitation period and a high risk of vision-threatening complications during and after surgery, the penetrating keratoplasty was typically indicated in advanced stages of FECD when a patient's vision became very poor. Treatment of corneal decompensation secondary to endothelial failure was revolutionized in the late 1990s[1] and was gradually

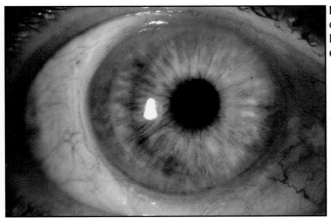

Figure 1-3. A patient with Fuchs's corneal endothelial dystrophy after Descemet's stripping automated endothelial keratoplasty.

replaced by posterior lamellar endothelial keratoplasty (most recently referred to as Descemet's stripping [automated] endothelial keratoplasty [DSEK or DSAEK]).[2] In 2007, 85% of patients who underwent a corneal transplant for corneal decompensation from endothelial failure in the United States underwent DSAEK. This procedure removes the diseased patient's corneal endothelium with Descemet's membrane and replaces it with a layer of donor cornea consisting of posterior corneal stroma, Descemet's membrane, and healthy endothelial cells. There are numerous advantages of DSAEK when compared to penetrating keratoplasty. Unlike penetrating keratoplasty, the surgery is performed through a small incision, which reduces the chance for catastrophic intraoperative subchoroidal hemorrhage during the surgery that can result in permanent loss of vision or the eye. The likelihood of such catastrophic bleeding with incidental ocular trauma after surgery is small compared to penetrating keratoplasty. Furthermore, the vision recovery after DSAEK is faster and superior to the vision recovery after penetrating keratoplasty. Patients typically reach near full recovery of vision within 1 month after DSAEK (Figure 1-3). The best-corrected visual acuity ranges between 20/20 and 20/40 in most patients, and the amount of surgically induced postoperative astigmatism is minimal compared to penetrating keratoplasty. Moreover, unlike penetrating keratoplasty, DSAEK does not lead to ocular surface disturbance, which typically contributes to a decrease in vision and prolonged vision recovery. On the other hand, the long-term data on endothelial cell count after DSAEK compare favorably to those seen after penetrating keratoplasty.[3]

Most recently, attempts to further improve vision after DSAEK have been made by Descemet's membrane endothelial keratoplasty (DMEK). The donor tissue in DMEK, unlike in DSAEK, has no or very little corneal stroma adhering to the Descemet's membrane. Preliminary data suggest that visual acuity after DMEK is superior to that seen after DSAEK, with 26% of patients achieving 20/20 and 63% achieving 20/25 or better, however, the trade-off is significantly increased donor harvesting failure, primary failure, and donor dislocations.[4]

References

1. Melles GRJ, Eggink FAGJ, Lander F, et al. A surgical technique for posterior lamellar keratoplasty. *Cornea.* 1998;17:618-626.
2. Gorovoy MS. Descemet-stripping automated endothelial keratoplasty. *Cornea.* 2006;25:879-881.

3. Price MO, Price FW. Endothelial cell density after Descemet's stripping endothelial keratoplasty: influencing factors and 2-year trend. *Ophthalmology.* 2008;115:857-865.
4. Price MO, Giebel AW, Fairchild KM, Price FW. Descemet membrane endothelial keratoplasty: prospective multicenter study of visual and refractive outcomes and endothelial survival. *Ophthalmology.* In press.

I AM SEEING A 64-YEAR-OLD FEMALE FOR CATARACT EVALUATION. THE SLIT-LAMP EXAMINATION IS SIGNIFICANT FOR ANTERIOR BASEMENT MEMBRANE DYSTROPHY AFFECTING THE VISUAL AXIS AND 2+ NUCLEAR SCLEROSIS OF THE LENS IN BOTH EYES. HOW SHOULD I MANAGE THIS PATIENT?

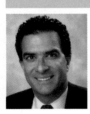

Sadeer B. Hannush, MD

It is important for the clinician to determine the contribution of both the corneal dystrophy and the cataract to the patient's visual compromise.

Anterior basement membrane dystrophy (ABMD) is the most common corneal dystrophy, with a predilection for women over men. The clinical appearance may vary and has been described extensively in the ophthalmic literature over the past century. *Map-dot, fingerprint, mare's tail* (Figure 2-1), and *Cogan's dystrophy* are terms used to describe this entity. Histopathologically, a thickened layer of epithelium is recognized together with reduplication of the epithelial basement membrane and entrapment of debris in cyst-like structures. In clinical practice, we encounter 2 presentations of ABMD: pain, photophobia, and tearing usually associated with the recurrent erosion syndrome manifestation of ABMD (discussed in a different chapter of this text) and decreased visual acuity associated with an irregular corneal surface overlying the pupillary aperture.

Figure 2-1. Cornea with anterior basement membrane dystrophy manifesting as "mare's tail."

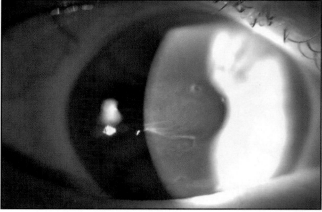

Work-Up and Treatment

Corneal topography may be an invaluable tool in evaluating the contribution of the basement membrane dystrophy to the patient's blurred vision. Irregular mires and an increased surface regularity index (SRI) usually imply that the surface is a significant contributor to the visual compromise. This may be further confirmed with a rigid gas-permeable (RGP) contact lens diagnostic evaluation. If the patient's vision improves significantly with a RGP lens, the cataract is not the main factor in the patient's poor vision, and cataract surgery should not be rushed into. Moreover, intraocular lens implant power calculations are likely to be inaccurate in the setting of inaccurate keratometry measurements.

In the preceding scenario, consideration should be given to treating the basement membrane dystrophy prior to cataract surgery. The patient is counseled in the following manner: she is advised that treatment of the basement membrane dystrophy may improve the vision enough to delay or obviate the need for cataract surgery. Moreover, treatment will likely create a smooth corneal surface, allowing accurate calculation of intraocular lens implant power, should the resultant vision after treatment of the basement membrane dystrophy be inadequate and a decision made to proceed with cataract surgery. With an irregular surface, any implant power calculation is an estimate at best.

If, on the other hand, the computerized corneal topography mires are relatively smooth, and there is minimal improvement in vision with a RGP contact lens, the surgeon may determine that the contribution of the basement membrane dystrophy to the patient's vision is minimal and may decide to proceed with cataract surgery alone. Implant power calculation may be carried out using the surgeon's technique of choice. The patient should still be counseled that vision after cataract surgery might not be crisp because of the corneal dystrophy and surgery might not result in spectacle independence.

When ABMD is visually significant, treatment usually consists of a superficial keratectomy. We favor a dull rounded or crescent knife to remove the central 5 to 6 mm of corneal epithelium overlying the pupillary aperture (Figure 2-2). The epithelial layer usually cleaves easily off of the basement membrane. It is very important to then deliberately remove the irregular, and frequently redundant, basement membrane until Bowman's layer is recognized with its characteristic sheen (Figure 2-3). The same keratectomy/epitheliectomy

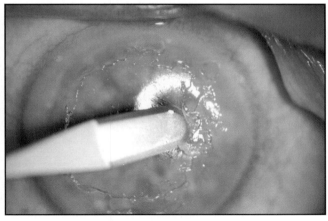

Figure 2-2. Superficial keratectomy removing the epithelium and basement membrane, baring Bowman's layer.

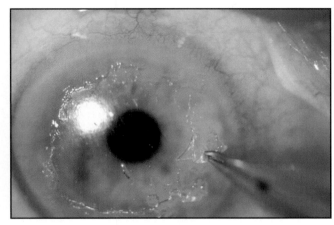

Figure 2-3. Peeling off basement membrane with forceps after epithelial removal. This photo demonstrates the sheen of Bowman's layer after the keratectomy.

may be accomplished with 20% ethanol as long as meticulous attention is given to removal of the abnormal basement membrane. Importantly, a diamond-dusted burr is not required in this setting. Because eliminating recurrent erosions is not the focus of treatment, roughening up Bowman's layer to improve adherence is not required (unnecessary diamond-dusted burr polishing of Bowman's layer may result in some fibrosis and visually significant haze). In the same vein, antifibrosis treatment with mitomycin is not necessary. Moreover, there is no real role for excimer laser phototherapeutic keratectomy in the treatment of ABMD in the absence of recurrent erosions. A therapeutic bandage contact lens is placed (eg, Acuvue Oasys). The patient is started on a topical steroid, nonsteroidal anti-inflammatory agent, and fluoroquinolone antibiotic, as is the custom with most surface procedures. Re-epithelialization usually takes place over the next 3 to 7 days. The bandage contact lens is then removed, the topical nonsteroidal anti-inflammatory agent and antibiotic discontinued, and the steroid tapered rapidly. A couple of weeks later, the patient is re-evaluated, visual acuity is remeasured, and computerized corneal topography is repeated. If the patient is pleased with her resultant vision, the endpoint of treatment is achieved. Otherwise, consideration may be given to proceeding with cataract surgery. Implant power calculation may be carried out using the technique preferred by the surgeon. We currently employ interferometry with the Zeiss IOLMaster.

The availability of premium IOL technology and the heightened expectations among patients and surgeons alike of excellent postoperative vision, unaided by spectacle or contact lens correction, necessitate paying extra attention to detail, specifically the identification of contributors other than the cataract to visual compromise. Optimization of the ocular surface including the preoperative treatment of mild forms of ABMD becomes very important.

Summary

Corneal ABMD is most commonly responsible for 2 clinical presentations:
1. Painful corneal erosions
2. Visual compromise

The ophthalmic literature is replete with articles describing techniques for the treatment and prevention of recurrent corneal erosions. These techniques most commonly employ a diamond-dusted burr[1,2] or excimer laser phototherapeutic keratectomy[2] to improve epithelial adherence after keratectomy, presumably by creating a mild inflammatory response and subclinical scar. When ABMD manifests as visual compromise alone without painful erosions, only removal of the corneal epithelium and underlying basement membrane is necessary. This may be achieved with a blade or with diluted ethanol. No adjuvant therapy with a diamond-dusted burr or laser is required. After Dr. Buxton's initial articles in the 1980s,[3,4] review of the literature did not reveal an article that specifically addresses this entity.

References

1. Wong VW, Chi SC, Lam DS. Diamond burr polishing for recurrent corneal erosions: results from a prospective randomized controlled trial. *Cornea*. 2009;28(2):152-156.
2. Sridhar MS, Rapuano CJ, Cosar CB, Cohen EJ, Laibson PR. Phototherapeutic keratectomy versus diamond burr polishing of Bowman's membrane in the treatment of recurrent corneal erosions associated with anterior basement membrane dystrophy. *Ophthalmology*. 2003;110(9):1855.
3. Buxton JN, Fox ML. Superficial epithelial keratectomy in the treatment of epithelial basement membrane dystrophy: a preliminary report. *Arch Ophthalmol*. 1983;101(3):392-395.
4. Buxton JN, Constad WH. Superficial epithelial keratectomy in the treatment of epithelial basement membrane dystrophy. *Cornea*. 1987;6(4):292-297.

A 62-Year-Old Male With No History of Ocular Surgery Complains of Blurry Vision in One Eye. The Exam Shows Diffuse Corneal Stromal Edema. How Should I Work Up and Treat This Patient?

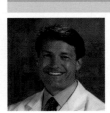

Anthony J. Aldave, MD

Unilateral corneal edema in the absence of prior intraocular surgery or dystrophic corneal endothelial changes in the contralateral eye is uncommon. However, it is important for ophthalmologists to be able to assemble a list of potential diagnoses in order to perform the appropriate diagnostic procedures and make the correct diagnosis. Potential diagnoses include idiopathic conditions such as iridocorneal endothelial syndrome; infectious or postinfectious conditions such as previous anterior uveitis and herpetic disciform endotheliitis, tears of Descemet's membrane secondary to forceps injury during birth, blunt trauma, congenital glaucoma or corneal ectasia; or dystrophic conditions such as nonguttate Fuchs' endothelial corneal dystrophy (FECD)[1] and posterior polymorphous corneal dystrophy (PPCD) (Figure 3-1).

Evaluation

The differentiation between the various causes of unilateral corneal edema begins with a careful history. Conditions such as forceps injury or congenital glaucoma, resulting in Descemet's rupture, should be identified during the history even before slit-lamp

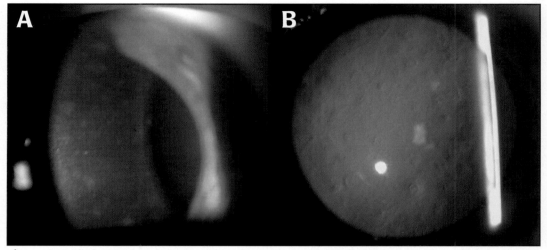

Figure 3-1. Slit-lamp photomicrographs of a patient with PPCD, demonstrating diffusely distributed endothelial opacities seen on direct (A) and indirect illumination (B).

examination is performed. Episodes of recurrent photophobia, decreased vision, and conjunctival injection would be consistent with recurrent anterior uveitis or herpetic keratouveitis, the diagnoses of which would be supported by a history of previous use of topical steroids and mydriatics. A family history of a corneal abnormality or transplantation would suggest a dominantly inherited corneal dystrophy, such as FECD or PPCD, which is also associated with an increased rate of abdominal wall hernias.[2]

Slit-lamp examination would be directed to evaluate for findings associated with the aforementioned potential diagnoses. The amount and distribution of the corneal edema may indicate the cause: axially distributed edema associated with FECD, localized edema associated with disciform keratitis and tears of Descemet's membrane, and the often diffuse edema associated with iridocorneal endothelial syndrome. Tears of Descemet's membrane, endothelial bands and vesicles, and keratic precipitates can obviously define the cause of the corneal edema but may be obscured by overlying stromal edema. While an anterior chamber reaction and posterior synechiae are commonly found in the setting of iritis, peripheral anterior synechiae, pupillary irregularity, iris nodules or atrophy, and elevated intraocular pressure (IOP) may be associated with either iritis or iridocorneal endothelial syndrome (Figure 3-2). The absence of photophobia, conjunctival injection, and an anterior chamber reaction in the latter aids in its differentiation from an inflammatory or infectious process.

Corneal pachymetry is part of the standard evaluation of all patients with corneal edema, primarily for management rather than diagnostic decision making. Specular microscopy is often not able to adequately visualize the corneal endothelium in the setting of stromal edema, and thus confocal microscopy may be required to estimate endothelial cell density and detect buried drusen associated with FECD and morphologic abnormalities associated with PPCD. If confocal microscopy is not available, high-resolution anterior segment imaging devices such as ultrasound biomicroscopy and optical coherence tomography may be used to detect tears of Descemet's membrane in cases

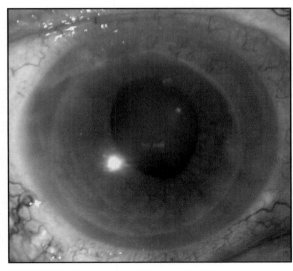

Figure 3-2. Slit-lamp photomicrograph of a patient following DSEK for unilateral corneal edema secondary to iridocorneal endothelial (ICE) syndrome. Note the vertical elongation of the pupil, secondary to peripheral anterior synechiae associated with ICE syndrome.

in which such tears are not visible by slit-lamp biomicroscopy due to significant stromal edema. While the corneal endothelium in the contralateral eye may appear normal by slit-lamp biomicroscopy, specular microscopic imaging may reveal the aforementioned dystrophic changes associated with FECD[1] and PPCD and has been reported to be abnormal in patients with ICE syndrome.[3]

While corneal topographic imaging in the involved eye may not be reliable in the setting of significant epithelial or stromal edema, it may detect or exclude a subclinical corneal ectatic disorder in the contralateral eye, providing evidence for or against a break of Descemet's membrane associated with a corneal ectatic disorder as the cause of the unilateral corneal edema.

The genetic basis of FECD remains to be elucidated, but the genetic basis of PPCD has been identified in approximately one third of affected families, providing a means to definitively confirm a presumptive clinical diagnosis.[2]

Management

While the management of visually significant corneal edema is nearly always surgical, medical management in the form of topical steroid therapy is the primary means of treatment for several causes of reversible corneal edema, such as herpetic disciform keratitis and iritis. Lowering of the IOP with topical glaucoma agents is indicated in cases of elevated IOP, even if only marginally elevated, to improve marginal endothelial cell function. In the absence of a corneal ectatic disorder or corneal scarring, in which case a penetrating keratoplasty would be indicated, the treatment of choice would be an endothelial keratoplasty. Histopathologic examination of the excised corneal button or Descemet's membrane would likely reveal the cause of the corneal edema, if not identified prior to surgery.

References

1. Abbott RL, Fine BS, Webster RG Jr, et al. Specular microscopic and histologic observations in nonguttate corneal endothelial degeneration. *Ophthalmology.* 1981;88:788-800.
2. Aldave AJ, Yallore VS, Yu F, et al. Posterior polymorphous corneal dystrophy is associated with TCF8 gene mutations and abdominal hernia. *Am J Med Genet A.* 2007;143:2549-2556.
3. Kupfer C, Kaiser-Kupfer MI, Datiles M, McCain L. The contralateral eye in the iridocorneal endothelial (ICE) syndrome. *Ophthalmology.* 1983;90:1343-1350.

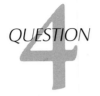

A Patient Has Irritation in Her Nonseeing Eye. The Exam Shows Mildly Inflamed Conjunctiva and Diffuse Corneal Epithelial and Stromal Edema With Large Bullae. What Should I Recommend?

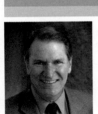

Mark A. Terry, MD

The treatment of painful pseudophakic bullous keratopathy (PBK) in a blind eye presents considerations that may be different from when the visual potential is light perception or better. In eyes that have had multiple surgeries producing the PBK and blindness, the goal is not visual restoration but pain relief and cosmetic acceptability. In addition, visualization by the ophthalmologist of the anterior chamber and optic nerve may not be a priority as it is in the seeing eye. Extensive discussion with the patient regarding individual outcome desires, reasonable goals, and expectations prior to any treatment should be the first step in the therapy.

Medical Therapy

The goal of pain relief cannot be achieved without resolution of the blistered surface. Use of a bandage contact lens (BCL) provides relief but may take months for secondary scarring of the bullae to provide a final resolution, and the danger of secondary bacterial or fungal infection is always present in this setting. Nonetheless, a BCL can provide temporary relief, and, with proper monitoring, months of relief can be achieved until a definitive surgical procedure is performed. Low-dose topical steroids with pulsed fluoroquinolone antibiotic coverage can concurrently be applied to reduce the discomfort of inflammation, but, once again, close monitoring of the eye is paramount. When the intraocular pressure (IOP) is above 20, I may start a beta-blocker or other glaucoma medication to lower the IOP and thereby reduce the force pressure pushing fluid into the cornea, which on occasion can also minimize bullae formation. Finally, in the absence of a BCL, the liberal use of hyperosmotic ointments/solutions such as 5% sodium chloride can reduce the size of the blisters, and the lubrication can reduce friction pain from the lid margin while blinking. Once again, all of these medical measures are temporary until either the natural course of the condition causes surface scarring to eliminate the pain or a definitive surgical procedure is accomplished.

Surgical Therapy

Surgical therapy is directed at either destroying or covering the sensory nerves to eliminate pain or restoring the endothelial function to eliminate the source of the PBK.

CONJUNCTIVAL FLAP SURGERY

If there is a sufficient amount of bulbar and fornix conjunctiva, my preference for the treatment of PBK in a no light perception (NLP) eye is the application of a Gunderson conjunctival flap.[1] The easiest and most abundant source of tissue for the flap is superior, but if this area is scarred from glaucoma surgery, the inferior bulbar and fornix conjunctiva can be mobilized. Complete removal, limbus to limbus, of the epithelium is performed, and a bridge flap anchored at the 3 and 9 o'clock positions can be sutured into position with vicryl or nylon 10-0 sutures at the limbus. I often perform a very shallow keratectomy at the peripheral limbus for even stronger long-term adhesion of the flap. For best cosmetic results, the flap should be made as thin as possible and button-holes are completely avoided. In cases where the anterior chamber needs to be viewed by the clinician (eg, chronic uveitis eyes, tumor resection eyes), a vertical incision at 200-µm depth can be made superiorly in the midperipheral cornea, a centrally adjacent 1-mm strip of superficial stroma can be excised, and the superior edge of the Gunderson flap can be sewn to the surface incision edge. In this manner, the flap often covers all of the painful bullae sites but leaves the peripheral superior cornea clear for viewing the intraocular structures. Gunderson flaps can be combined with lid tarsorrhaphy, BCL, or patching to ensure initial flap epithelial health. Antibiotics and steroids are used 4 times daily until the sutures are removed or dissolved, usually within 2 to 3 weeks. Comfort with a conjunctival flap is usually immediate, and a well-created flap can yield excellent cosmetic results at 6 months or earlier. Furthermore, once healed, the Gunderson flap patient requires minimal clinical monitoring, little or no medication, and, if unsatisfied with the cosmesis of the flap itself, becomes a candidate for a scleral shell prosthesis.

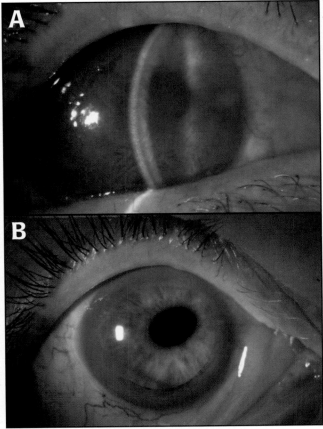

Figure 4-1. Preoperative photo of eye with severe traumatic painful bullous keratopathy (A). Post-operative photo of the same eye 6 months later with clear endothelial keratoplasty graft and relief of pain (B).

SURFACE SCARRING SURGERY

In PBK eyes with multiple surgeries, especially retinal and glaucoma surgeries, the bulbar conjunctiva is frequently so severely scarred that conjunctival flap surgery is difficult or impossible. Acceleration of surface scarring for pain relief can be achieved by the scraping of the epithelial bullae followed by micropuncture, shallow lamellar keratoplasty (with a rough diamond burr, blade, or femtosecond laser phototherapeutic keratectomy), or application of diathermy.[2] In consideration of the health care costs and ease of treatment, I prefer the diamond burr procedure. For all of these therapies, epithelial resurfacing is crucial, and I recommend the addition of human amniotic membrane coverage to reduce inflammation and promote fast re-epithelialization. The patient also must be informed of the possible acute increase in pain following these procedures, and appropriate topical and systemic medical pain management should be performed. In addition, some bullae can recur, and a second therapeutic application may be required.

ENDOTHELIAL KERATOPLASTY

In the setting of PBK and relatively normal conjunctiva and iris anatomy, the best cosmetic result and full relief of pain can be achieved with endothelial keratoplasty (EK) surgery (Figure 4-1).[3] As an intraocular surgery, the preoperative risk counseling of the patient obviously is different, and the extended time for postoperative medications and frequency of clinic visits needs to be thoroughly discussed. The largest diameter EK graft should be used, but even an 8.0-mm graft offers extensive pain relief, as peripheral limbal bullae are often asymptomatic and eventually will spontaneously scar over. The relative health-care costs involved with EK surgery versus surface surgery need to be weighed as does the effect on the eye bank community of using a precious resource of donor corneal tissue for a nonseeing eye. However, in selected cases, an EK can succeed in the primary goal of pain elimination, with the added benefit of intraocular structure visualization by the clinician, and a near normal appearance of the blind eye.

References

1. Nichols BD, Anjema CM. Conjunctival flaps. In: Krachmer J, Mannis M, Holland E, eds. *Cornea*. 2nd ed. Philadelphia, PA: Elsevier; 2005:1763-1771.
2. Rich LF. Corneal surgery for ocular surface disease. In: Krachmer J, Mannis M, Holland E, eds. *Cornea*. 2nd ed. Philadelphia, PA: Elsevier; 2005:1729-1733.
3. Terry MA, Shamie N, Chen ES, Hoar KL, Friend DF. Endothelial keratoplasty: a simplified technique to minimize graft dislocation, iatrogenic graft failure and pupillary block. *Ophthalmology*. 2008;115:1179-1186.

A PATIENT WITH RECURRENT EROSION SYNDROME IS COMPLAINING OF IRRITATION AND PAIN IN THE RIGHT EYE THAT TYPICALLY WAKES HER UP EARLY IN THE MORNING. WHAT SHOULD I DO?

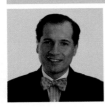

Dimitri T. Azar, MD
(co-authored with Kristina Thomas, MD)

Recurrent erosion syndrome (RES) is a common condition characterized by one or more episodes of breakdown of the corneal epithelium due to adhesion abnormalities between the corneal epithelium, basement membrane, and the underlying stroma. Symptoms include repeated episodes of pain, photophobia, tearing, and difficulty opening the eyes upon awakening.

The intensity of symptoms and the rate of recurrence can vary greatly between patients. Some patients may experience only minor symptoms every few months or years. Other patients may have frequent, severe, debilitating symptoms that persist for days and are often associated with areas of loose epithelium that move with every blink, causing persistent pain.

Clinical history and careful slit-lamp examination are essential in the diagnosis of RES. A history of recurrent episodes of pain, tearing, and/or difficulty opening the eyes upon awakening, as described by this patient, is characteristic. In addition, the patient should always be asked about a history of trauma to the affected eye. On slit-lamp examination, often only subtle signs of RES remain; nevertheless, anything from a gross epithelial defect to subtle intra-epithelial pseudocysts can be seen.[1] Examination of both eyes using a broad, angled slit beam, with and without fluorescein instillation, can help to identify the problem areas. I find it beneficial to dilate the pupils and then to examine the cornea under retroillumination, which often helps to identify the subtle signs of epithelial basement membrane dystrophy or previous areas of erosions. In addition, by applying minimal pressure to the epithelium through the eyelid, areas of wrinkling can identify loosely adherent epithelium or abnormal areas.

Some patients with RES will not have any findings upon presentation, and the diagnosis is made only by the clinical history. If the diagnosis is in question, however, the patient should be instructed to return during the next episode, while the epithelium is still abnormal. In addition, other etiologies of RES should be explored. Prior trauma to the affected eye and epithelial basement membrane dystrophy are the 2 most common causes of RES[1]; however, many other conditions are associated with the syndrome. For example, floppy eyelids, lagophthalmos, keratoconjunctivitis sicca, and diabetes mellitus can be causes of RES and therefore should be explored.[2]

The pathology of RES is not completely understood. Microscopy of post-traumatic recurrent erosion corneas has shown partial absence of basement membrane as well as loss of hemidesmosomes.[1,2] In addition, areas of discontinued and redundant basement membrane, along with a decreased number of anchoring fibrils, were found.

Treatment Options

The goal of treatment for RES is to increase the adherence of the epithelium to the underlying basement membrane and stroma. We use a step ladder approach for the treatment of RES, starting with hyperosmotic drops and ointments. We first recommend using sodium chloride 5% drops during the day and sodium chloride 5% ointment at night. The logic for using hyperosmotic agents to treat RES is based on the decreased evaporation and relative hypotonicity of the tear film at night.[2] The hyperosmotic ointment also serves as a lubricant to prevent erosions during sleep and upon eyelid opening. Hyperosmotic drops are used during the daytime to reduce edema, again hoping to promote adhesions between the epithelium and the underlying basement membrane and stroma. This treatment should be attempted for 12 to 15 weeks to allow proper reformation of adhesion complexes.[1] Patients may be quick to discontinue treatment once they feel they are "cured"; therefore, it is important to educate patients about the importance of continuing treatment as planned.

If hyperosmotic agents fail to prevent the patient from having recurrent erosions, we place a bandage contact lens. A contact lens that is safe for continuous wear, such as CIBA Vision's Focus Night and Day, is ideal. The lens will provide symptomatic relief while promoting healing of the epithelium and adhesion complexes, especially if any eyelid abnormalities exist. A prophylactic antibiotic drop should be used with or without the continuation of the hyperosmotic drop. Recent studies have also shown the benefit of using scleral contact lenses when RES is secondary to ocular surface disorders.[2] In any case, the contact lens should be placed for 3 months, as remodeling of the basement membrane requires a minimum of 12 weeks.

If the erosions recur after the contact lens is removed, more aggressive treatments are required to prevent recurrences. The first and least invasive surgical treatment available is debridement. This procedure can be performed at the slit lamp, under topical anesthesia, using a cotton-tip applicator or blunt spatula to remove the loosely adherent layers of epithelium. The goal is to allow the epithelium to heal and hopefully form normal adhesion complexes. The disadvantage of this procedure is that it does not directly address the underlying problems of adhesion.[1,2] In order to promote normal epithelial adhesion, a diamond burr can then be used to polish Bowman's layer after debridement.[3] If the area of recurrent erosions involves the central visual axis, the entire epithelium is removed except a 1- to 2-mm peripheral rim of epithelium, and the surface is then polished using even, circular movements to avoid creating irregular astigmatism. A bandage contact lens and topical nonsteroidal anti-inflammatory agents are used for comfort after the procedure.

Another technique often used by ophthalmologists to treat RES is anterior stromal puncture, first described by McLean and colleagues in 1986.[1,2] Using a 25-gauge needle, punctures are placed through affected areas of loose epithelium and into the anterior stroma about 0.5 mm apart. The treated area should extend at least 1 mm into the normal epithelium bordering the affected area. The rationale behind this treatment is that breaks in Bowman's layer will incite scar formation and thus adhesions between epithelium, basement membrane, and stroma. The main disadvantage of this procedure is that if performed in the central visual axis, it may induce scarring and irregular astigmatism.

In the event that other treatments fail, phototherapeutic keratectomy is a safe and effective treatment for unmanageable cases of RES. Studies report the success rate ranging from 74% to 100%, with erosions secondary to trauma having a higher success rate than those due to dystrophies.[4] Microscopic studies have shown that new basement membrane and hemidesmosomes form by 2 weeks after photoablation; however, anchoring fibrils, hemidesmosomes, and basal lamina can take up to 15 months to stabilize.[1,2,5] Therefore, it is essential the patient be followed for at least 15 months before considering the treatment a success. The patient's epithelium is scraped mechanically prior to excimer treatment, which is limited to 2 to 8 μm in depth across the central and paracentral cornea. The main postoperative complication is a refractive shift toward hyperopia, which is reduced by using small ablation depths of less than 5 μm.

References

1. Ramamurthi S, Rahman MQ, Dutton GN, Ramaesh K. Pathogenesis, clinical features and management of recurrent erosions. *Eye.* 2006;20:635-644.
2. Das S, Seitz B. Recurrent corneal erosion syndrome. *Surv Ophthalmol.* 2008;53(1):3-15.
3. Wong WY, Chi SC, Lam DS. Diamond burr polishing for recurrent corneal erosions: results from a prospective randomized controlled trial. *Cornea.* 2009;28:152-156.
4. Baryla J, Pan YI, Hodge WG. Long-term efficacy of phototherapeutic keratectomy on recurrent corneal erosion syndrome. *Cornea.* 2006;10:1150-1152.
5. Fountain TR, de la Cruz Z, Green WR, Stark WJ, Azar DT. Reassembly of corneal epithelial adhesion structures after excimer laser keratectomy in humans. *Arch Ophthalmol.* 1994;112(7):967-972.

A PATIENT WITH A FILTERING BLEB COMPLAINS OF DISCOMFORT IN THE EYE. THE BLEB IS PROLAPSING ONTO THE CORNEA AND AN AREA OF STROMAL THINNING AND EPITHELIAL STAINING WITH FLUORESCEIN IS ADJACENT TO THE BLEB. WHAT IS THE OPTIMAL MANAGEMENT?

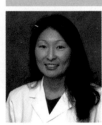

Sonia H. Yoo, MD
(co-authored with Mohamed Abou Shousha, MD)

A successful filtering surgery should not only achieve long-term reduction of intraocular pressure but it should also have a minimal impact on the ocular surface and patient comfort. The morphology of the filtration bleb is an important factor to achieve those aims. Ideally, the bleb should be diffuse with minimal impact on the ocular surface. However, a large filtering bleb could encroach on the cornea and cause corneal dellen. A dellen in most instances is a benign lesion. However, in severe cases, a corneal dellen, if untreated, can lead to a descemetocele and corneal perforation.[1]

The term *dellen* is derived from the German word for "dents" and refers to saucer-shaped depressions of the cornea most commonly at the periphery. The lesion occurs at or near the limbus adjacent to raised abnormal tissue on the bulbar conjunctiva that prevents the eyelid from adequately resurfacing the cornea with tears during blinking. Localized interruption of the tear film occurs, leading to desiccation of the epithelium and subepithelial tissue. This can also cause the underlying sclera to become markedly thinned and translucent, forming a scleral dellen.

Clinically, a dellen is seen as a saucer-like corneal thinning just anterior to the limbus. Typically, the corneal epithelium remains intact (Figure 6-1), but in severe cases there may be de-epithelialization. The epithelium exhibits punctate irregularities overlying a thinned area of dehydrated corneal stroma. Fluorescein pools in these depressions but does not stain the stroma. They cause mild discomfort and should be treated with lubrication and close observation.

Dellen have been observed in association with filtering blebs (see Figure 6-1) as well as pingueculae, pterygia, rectus muscle surgery, bullous subconjunctival hemorrhage and injections, limbal tumors, and cataract surgery.

The incidence of dellen after filtering glaucoma surgery was reported in several studies to be between 2% and 30% and in most instances adjacent to large cystic blebs. The wide variation in incidence is probably due to differences in the surgical techniques and thus different sizes of the resulting bleb. The rate of dellen also was reported to be higher in superonasal blebs than superotemporal and least in superior blebs. This could be explained by the observation that filtering bleb dysesthesia occurs more commonly in superonasal blebs.[2]

Dellen with a bleb should not be confused with other causes of peripheral corneal thinning or ulcerative keratitis. Dellen are localized and are always adjacent to the causative conjunctival or limbal elevated lesion. Obviously, infectious infiltrates and ulcers have to be ruled out. Slit-lamp examination of a dellen should not reveal any infiltrates. Typically, the eye is very quiet, and the patient complains only of mild discomfort.

In the setting of a filtering glaucoma surgery with adjunctive use of antimetabolites such as mitomycin C, corneal and conjunctival toxicity should be considered. However, such cases will manifest with punctate epithelial erosions, primary conjunctival wound leaks in addition to the corneal epithelial defects. Worth mentioning are eyes with limbal stem cell deficiency that could also present with persistent epithelial defects. This condition should be differentiated from dellen by the presence of conjunctivalization, surface irregularities, and vascularization of the cornea. Terrien's marginal degeneration could also be confused with a dellen as it produces a quiet peripheral corneal thinning, leaving the epithelium intact. However, that condition is often bilateral and first presents as a peripheral corneal haze that, over time, exhibits a slowly progressive peripheral corneal thinning with a sloping central edge that spares the limbus. A severe dellen that is de-epithelialized with severe stromal thinning and melting could be confused with other causes of peripheral ulcerative keratitis such as connective tissue diseases, Mooren's ulcer, rosacea keratitis, or severe dry eye. Those causes have to be ruled out from the differential diagnosis.

Management

Treatment of dellen associated with filtering blebs may be complicated by the need to preserve the functioning bleb as opposed to the need to heal the cornea. Medical treatment includes aggressive lubrication with artificial tears and aqueous suppressants. Lubrication in most instances cures the dellen by hydrating the tissue and re-expanding the locally compacted stromal lamellae. Aqueous suppressants could help to decrease the

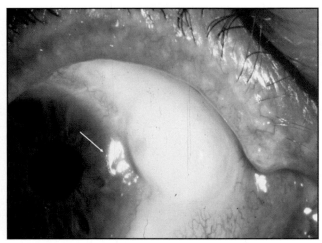

Figure 6-1. Painful dellen (arrow) in front of an exposed elevated bleb. (Photo courtesy of Paul Palmberg, MD, Bascom Palmer Eye Institute.)

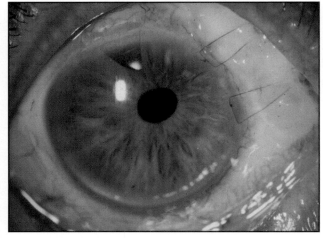

Figure 6-2. Two 9-0 mattress compression sutures were anchored in clear cornea in front of the bleb and anchored in deep Tenon's capsule behind, and the knot was rotated into the cornea. (Photo courtesy of Paul Palmberg, MD, Bascom Palmer Eye Institute.)

size of the bleb, eliminating the causative factor. In cases of persistent dellen or if there is any sign of de-epithelialization, topical steroids, which are usually prescribed to guard against scarring and failure of the bleb, have to be tapered or discontinued according to the severity of the dellen. In general, blebs become flatter over time, and many dellen with blebs, unlike dellen associated with other limbal elevations, do well without intervention and with only conservative treatment. However, in cases with intractable pain caused by dellen, fluctuation in vision caused by tearing and corneal drying, or persistent dellen with stromal melting, intervention to eliminate the causative factor is warranted. Many techniques have been described for bleb reduction and bleb repair such as trichloroacetic acid, compression suture (Figures 6-2 and 6-3), and autologous blood injection. Surgical intervention carries a risk of inducing scarring and failure of the bleb, and thus it should be reserved only for severe cases that are unresponsive to medical therapy.[3,4]

Figure 6-3. Sutures were removed 14 days postoperatively. Intraocular pressure was 8 mm Hg. The bleb contour was changed. Dellen were gone and did not return. (Photo courtesy of Paul Palmberg, MD, Bascom Palmer Eye Institute.)

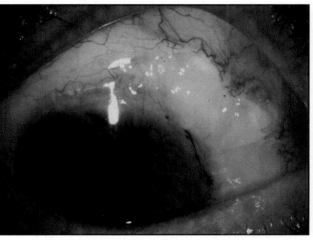

References

1. Baum JL, Mishima S, Boruchoff SA. On the nature of dellen. *Arch Ophthalmol*. 1968;79:657-662.
2. Budenz DL, Hoffman K, Zacchei A. Glaucoma filtering bleb dysesthesia. *Am J Ophthalmol*. 2001;131: 626-630.
3. La Borwit SE, Quigley HA, Jampel HD. Bleb reduction and bleb repair after trabeculectomy. *Ophthalmology*. 2000;107:712-718.
4. Haynes WL, Alward WL. Combination of autologous blood injection and bleb compression sutures to treat hypotony maculopathy. *J Glaucoma*. 1999;8:384-387.

A 63-Year-Old Male Complaining of Blurry Vision Has 360-Degree Peripheral Corneal Stromal Thinning and Conjunctivalization and Moderate Cataract in Both Eyes. Does He Need Surgery?

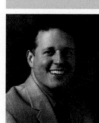

J. Bradley Randleman, MD

Peripheral corneal thinning represents a final common manifestation of degenerative corneal changes rather than a specific disease entity, and the diagnosis and management of this condition depends largely on patient history, symptoms, comorbidities, and severity at presentation. Peripheral corneal thinning can cause problems directly as well as confounding other ocular surgeries, especially cataract removal.

Differential Diagnosis

The differential diagnosis for peripheral corneal thinning is quite large; however, potential etiologies can be significantly narrowed by analyzing the specific location and distribution of the corneal thinning as well as evaluating the patient's overall health and comorbidities.[1] Due to its proximity to the limbal vasculature, the peripheral cornea is susceptible to vascular disease or inflammatory processes that generally spare the central cornea. Peripheral corneal thinning disorders can be categorized based on the presence or absence of neovascular changes.

The most common peripheral corneal thinning disorders without associated vascularization include furrow degeneration and pellucid marginal corneal degeneration (PMCD). Furrow degeneration is typically a bilateral, mild thinning process found in elderly patients with minimal associated symptoms. Thinning is circumferential but may be asymmetric, and no management is required. PMCD is characterized by a more localized peripheral corneal thinning, which usually presents inferiorly but can be located in any meridian (Figure 7-1).[2] PMCD is also bilateral but can be highly asymmetric and shares many characteristics with keratoconus, including overlapping topographic patterns. In contrast to furrow degeneration, corneal thinning can be extensive and visually debilitating in patients with PMCD. There is commonly high corneal astigmatism, and many patients require rigid gas-permeable contact lenses or corneal transplantation for visual rehabilitation.

The most common peripheral corneal thinning disorders with associated vascularization include Terrien's marginal degeneration and peripheral inflammatory conditions, including peripheral ulcerative keratitis related to blepharitis or systemic vasculitides, most commonly rheumatoid arthritis, and the ill-defined Mooren's ulcer.

Terrien's marginal degeneration represents a hybrid condition between peripheral disorders with and without neovascularization. While Terrien's almost invariably has some degree of neovascularization in its presentation (Figures 7-2 and 7-3), patients are usually asymptomatic or only minimally symptomatic, and inflammation is rarely seen. Similar to PCMD, Terrien's is usually relatively isolated in location[3]; however, it most commonly presents superiorly rather than inferiorly. Patients most commonly present with marked degrees of corneal astigmatism but rarely require any corneal surgery.

In contrast, other peripheral corneal disorders with neovascularization are associated with significant inflammation and usually severe symptoms, including redness, pain, photophobia, and occasionally discharge. Inflammatory peripheral thinning disorders often have chronic symptoms along with acute exacerbations (Figure 7-4).

Peripheral infiltrates are common during acute exacerbations, and it may be difficult to distinguish purely inflammatory processes from infectious processes. Infiltrates are especially common in blepharitis-related peripheral inflammatory conditions in the form of catarrhal ulcers or phlyctenules. Affected individuals may have rosacea with concomitant dermatologic findings. Systemic immunologic disease manifesting as peripheral corneal thinning is also highly symptomatic but less frequently associated with peripheral infiltrates. Mooren's ulcer, a unique inflammatory process, may be rapidly progressive and involve the entire cornea.

In this patient with bilateral diffuse thinning with associated neovascularization and a probable history of inflammation, the most likely diagnosis is either severe blepharitis or autoimmune disease.

Patient Work-Up and Management

For the majority of patients with peripheral corneal thinning, including those without neovascularization, minimal work-up beyond the routine slit-lamp examination is needed, and no systemic work-up is necessary. Corneal topography may be useful in characterizing the cause of the thinning and may be especially helpful in identifying the

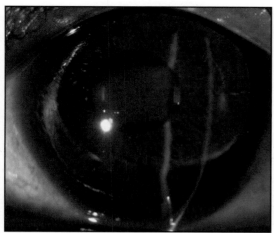

Figure 7-1. Pellucid marginal corneal degeneration. Note the significant inferior thinning visible in the slit-beam view of light.

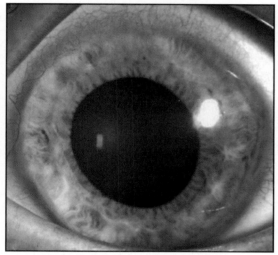

Figure 7-2. Terrien's marginal corneal degeneration. Note the peripheral corneal vascularization in the superior portion of the cornea. Despite this degree of vascularization, the eye is relatively quiet.

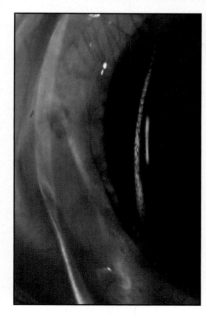

Figure 7-3. Terrien's marginal corneal degeneration. Close-up view of the peripheral cornea demonstrating significant peripheral thinning.

Figure 7-4. Peripheral cornea thinning with associated inflammation. Note the diffuse conjunctival inflammation and circumferential peripheral neovascularization with associated thinning.

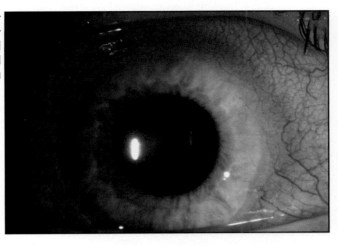

degree of irregular astigmatism, which will affect the success of visual correction with spectacles. Management for these conditions includes visual rehabilitation with either spectacles or contact lenses and monitoring for progression.

For patients with bilateral, relatively diffuse corneal thinning associated with inflammation, further investigation is necessary, and systemic work-up may prove valuable to identify patients with vasculitides and autoimmune processes, especially rheumatoid arthritis.

External and slit-lamp evaluation should identify blepharitis-related processes. Referral to a dermatologist may be necessary to treat other skin manifestations for patients with rosacea. Management includes the use of oral and topical tetracycline-related compounds, lid hygiene, and hot compresses to facilitate meibomian gland function. Additionally, tear film issues should be addressed with tear substitutes and topical cyclosporine as needed. During acute exacerbations, topical antibiotics and topical steroids may be needed but should be used judiciously.

If a systemic immune-related process is suspected, a thorough review of systems may help identify the underlying disease process. The full extent of the work-up will vary from patient to patient, but patient care is ideally coordinated with the patient's primary care physician with referral to a rheumatologist as needed.

The diagnosis of Mooren's ulcer is one of exclusion and should be made only after work-up has failed to identify any other cause for the inflammatory thinning. Pain is a common feature, and, in some patients, the corneal changes have a rapid progression. Management includes aggressive use of topical and systemic steroids and related medications.

For this patient, if external evaluation did not definitively identify blepharitis as the underlying cause for thinning, a systemic work-up and referral would be appropriate.

Indications for Corneal Surgery

Most patients with peripheral corneal thinning do not require surgical intervention. In rare cases of noninflammatory peripheral corneal thinning, severe, progressive corneal thinning may require lamellar keratoplasty to prevent or manage corneal perforations.

Corneal warpage in pellucid marginal corneal degeneration may progress to the point that penetrating keratoplasty is required for visual rehabilitation. These grafts are often challenging depending on the location of the thinnest region of the cornea and the overall integrity of the peripheral corneal tissue in the most affected region.

Inflammatory peripheral disease occasionally leads to corneal melts. These can also be managed with lamellar keratoplasty; however, the prognosis is guarded if the underlying inflammatory process cannot be medically controlled.

Corneal perforation is more commonly associated with Mooren's ulcer, and, again, the prognosis for this condition is guarded.

Considerations for Cataract Surgery

Alterations to normal surgical technique for cataract removal in patients with peripheral corneal thinning will depend on the etiology, location, and severity of thinning present. When considering wound location and construction, the area of thinning should be avoided. If the cause is noninflammatory, either clear cornea or scleral tunnel wounds should be effective. However, with inflammatory corneal thinning disorders, trauma to the conjunctiva should be avoided; these patients are better suited for clear corneal incisions that avoid areas of corneal thinning. Corneal melts have been reported with the use of topical nonsteroidal medications; thus, judicious use of topical anti-inflammatory medications is necessary to reduce the risk of corneal melts.

Many patients with peripheral corneal thinning will have induced corneal astigmatism. Because much of this astigmatism is irregular, astigmatism management is challenging. Limbal relaxing incisions (LRIs) are not advisable because the peripheral corneal thickness is less than normal and perforations at the time of LRI placement can occur. Further, there is significant potential to weaken an already thinned peripheral cornea and predispose it to increased risk of rupture from minimal trauma. Finally, LRIs can be somewhat unpredictable in normal corneas, and they are much more prone to inaccurate results in these abnormal corneas.

If the majority of the astigmatism is regular and the corneal changes have been stable, toric intraocular lens (IOL) implantation is a possible management strategy. However, patients should be counseled that their astigmatism may change over their lifetime and render the toric IOL relatively less effective over time.

Summary

Patients with peripheral corneal thinning represent a unique diagnostic and management challenge to the ophthalmologist. Care for these patients may require coordination with other physicians. Careful surgical planning at the time of cataract surgery is needed to maximize visual outcomes.

References

1. Stern GA. Peripheral corneal disease. In: Krachmer JH, Mannis MJ, Holland EJ (eds). *Cornea*. 2nd ed. New York, NY: Mosby; 2004:339-352.
2. Sridhar MS, Mahesh S, Bansal AK, et al. Pellucid marginal corneal degeneration. *Ophthalmology*. 2004; 111:1102-1107.
3. Guyer DR, Barraquer J, McDonnell PJ, Green WR. Terrien's marginal degeneration: clinicopathologic case reports. *Graefes Arch Clin Exp Ophthalmol*. 1987;225(1):19-27.

A Patient With Eye Irritation While Wearing Soft Contact Lenses Is Noted to Have White Elevated Nodules at the Limbus: Does She Need Surgery?

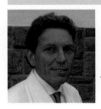

Thomas Kohnen, MD

Salzmann's nodular degeneration (SND) is a noninflammatory, slowly progressive degenerative disorder. SND is characterized by bluish-gray (or white) nodules that usually vary in number and are elevated above the corneal surface; sometimes, they are confluent. They occur either in the scarred cornea or at the edge of the transparent cornea with or without presence of vascularization. Many years elapse before SND causes loss of vision and requires surgery. The disease may be unilateral or bilateral, which suggests a careful exam of the second eye if SND is diagnosed in one eye. SND affects patients of various ages and different races. The disease displays a predilection for the female gender, so this case is very typical. SND can be associated with a history of ocular surface diseases (eg, phlyctenular keratitis, interstitial keratitis, vernal keratitis, trachoma, Thygeson superficial punctate keratitis, scarlet fever, measles, and keratoconjunctivitis). In other cases, however, there is no history of previous eye disease.

Diagnosis

SND will not be very frequent in general practice; more often, it will be seen by corneal specialists. Therefore, you should consider every single case very carefully. The first diagnostic instrument should always be an evaluation of the anterior segment with the slit lamp (Figure 8-1). Further, in vivo confocal microscopy has shown its applicability for diagnosis of SND by being correlated to histopathological findings.[1] Using in vivo confocal microscopy will give you important information about your patient's degree of SND and, thus, the required treatment.

Treatment

The etiology of the disease is unknown, and a spontaneous cure or remission has never been reported. Therefore, surgical treatment is the only option for improving the vision of patients with SND. Nodules can be successfully removed manually by superficial keratectomy provided the opacity is confined to the superficial layers of the cornea with or without subsequent phototherapeutic keratectomy (PTK) using an excimer laser.[2] In most instances, healing is rapid and visual disturbances decrease. Even without performance of PTK, rehabilitation and healing give a good result, but PTK may provide a more regular surface and therefore should be added to the surgical treatment. If the SND recurs, one should consider PTK as a possible treatment as well (Figure 8-2). Large nodules can extend deeply into the stroma. Such cases may require PTK or, in severe cases, lamellar or penetrating keratoplasty. Severin and Kirchhof reported superficial opacity of grafts 2.5 and 9 years after penetrating keratoplasty because of recurring SND.[3] Recurrence can also occur after surgical treatments like keratoplasty or PTK.

Postoperative Protocol

The usual postoperative medical therapy consists of artificial tears and antibiotic eye drops. Both should be applied until total healing of epithelium is achieved, followed by steroid eye drops up to 4 weeks after surgery. To prevent such recurrence, Bowers and colleagues applied mitomycin-C (MMC) after superficial keratectomy.[4] None of the patients treated in this manner suffered a recurrence of SND during a follow-up period of up to 4 years. However, MMC for prophylaxis of SND is an off-label use. I do not typically use MMC. If SND recurs, however, one should consider it as an option for retreatment.

Correction of Ametropia

One female patient with SND was +6.00 D prior to surgery. After epithelial removal and performance of PTK, the patient was emmetropic.[1] Because of the change in corneal refractive power induced by the nodules, refractive surgery should not be combined with SND treatment. It seems to me that SND causes very bad predictability in refractive surgery and, thus, should not be performed to avoid any risk of large under- or over-corrections.

Due to the irregular corneal surface, contact lens fitting will be difficult in patients still suffering from SND. One should not consider contact lens fitting prior to the treatment. However, after the treatment and complete wound healing, contact lenses may be fit.

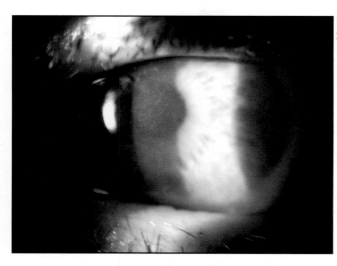

Figure 8-1. Slit-lamp examination of SND prior to treatment.

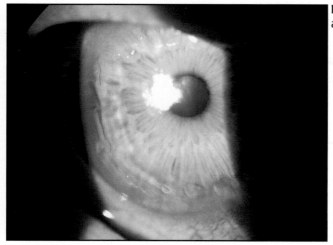

Figure 8-2. Slit-lamp examination after PTK.

It is important to schedule regular visits to control the contact lens fitting and the possible recurrence of SND afterwards. If there is any sign of contact lens intolerance, their use should be discontinued. One has to instruct patients very carefully to take out contact lenses in case of discomfort.

References

1. Meltendorf C, Buhren J, Bug R, Ohrloff C, Kohnen T. Correlation between clinical in vivo confocal microscopic and ex vivo histopathologic findings of Salzmann nodular degeneration. *Cornea.* 2006;25:734-738.
2. Das S, Langenbucher A, Pogorelov P, Link B, Seitz B. Long-term outcome of excimer laser phototherapeutic keratectomy for treatment of Salzmann's nodular degeneration. *J Cataract Refract Surg.* 2005;31:1386-1391.
3. Severin M, Kirchhof B. Recurrent Salzmann's corneal degeneration. *Graefes Arch Clin Exp Ophthalmol.* 1990;228:101-104.
4. Bowers PJ Jr, Price MO, Zeldes SS, Price FW Jr. Superficial keratectomy with mitomycin-C for the treatment of Salzmann's nodules. *J Cataract Refract Surg.* 2003;29:1302-1306.

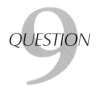

QUESTION **9**

A 22-YEAR-OLD FEMALE COMPLAINING OF BLURRY VISION IN ONE EYE HAS DEEP SECTORAL CORNEAL STROMAL NEOVASCULARIZATION WITH STROMAL INFILTRATE AND LIPID DEPOSITS IN THE CENTER OF THE CORNEA. HOW SHOULD I MANAGE THIS PATIENT?

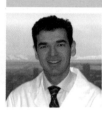

Majid Moshirfar, MD, FACS
(co-authored with JoAnn C. Chang, MD)

Corneal neovascularization (NV) is a potentially sight-threatening condition. However, if recognized and treated properly, patients can experience minimal loss of best-corrected visual acuity (BCVA). Corneal NV can occur at multiple corneal layers. Superficial corneal NV or vascular pannus is associated mainly with ocular surface disorders and contact lens wear. Corneal stromal NV is associated with inflammatory, infectious, traumatic, and contact lens wear and can be associated with necrosis, haze, thinning, and lipid keratopathy. Previous episodes of unilateral red, sore eyes; blurred vision; cold sores; and rashes may suggest herpetic etiology. Patients with herpetic stromal keratitis usually suffer from photophobia and irritated red eyes, as opposed to contact lens wearer who may be asymptomatic until the vision is decreased. Clinically, one should check for decreased corneal sensitivity, epithelial breakdown and staining, subepithelial haze (ghost scarring from previous herpetic epithelial keratitis), anterior chamber cell, keratic precipitates, and iris atrophy, which may suggest herpetic etiology. Unfortunately, herpetic interstitial keratitis with stromal NV can be associated with all or none of the additional clinical entities. If there is no history of contact lens wear, trauma, or concurrent ocular infection, I would treat this patient for presumed herpetic stromal keratitis.

Interstitial keratitis from syphilis was the most common cause of cornea stromal NV historically, but it is uncommon today. Findings like chorioretinal scarring and dental and bony malformations may be present. Other less common causes of stromal NV include mycobacterial, Lyme, parasitic (including acanthamoeba), Epstein-Barr virus, mumps, Cogan's syndrome, and other autoimmune diseases. History of recent illness, travel, skin lesions or rashes, and vestibuloauditory symptoms can assist you in narrowing your diagnosis.

This patient should be worked up based on history and clinical findings. Syphilis is diagnosed based on history, clinical findings, and serology treponemal and nontreponemal tests. Purified protein derivative (PPD) may be placed if the patient exhibits cough, fever, or night sweats or has had a recent incarceration or travel. Lyme titers and enzyme-linked immunosorbent assay (ELISA) may aid in diagnosis of Lyme disease. Herpetic stromal disease with an intact epithelium is typically immunologic; diagnosis will be based on history and clinical findings.

Treatment Options

Inflammation is usually involved in the pathogenesis of any stromal NV. The mainstay treatment is topical corticosteroids. Active infectious etiology must be ruled out before starting any topical steroid regimen. There are no strict guidelines for management of stromal NV; treatment should be individualized for each patient based on the level of inflammation. Some clinicians advocate not initiating corticosteroid therapy for early or mild stromal keratitis. For this young patient with a unilateral deep stromal NV, diffuse stromal infiltrate, and decreased vision, I would start with a significant strength topical corticosteroid (ie, prednisolone acetate 1% or difluprednate 0.05%) with adequate frequency to suppress the inflammation. The potential sequelae from herpetic stromal keratitis are sufficient enough for me to start her on concurrent oral antivirals. It is important to gradually taper the corticosteroid to prevent recurrence. For some patients, especially ones with HSV stromal keratitis, lower-dose topical corticosteroids (ie, prednisolone acetate 0.125% or fluorometholone 0.1%) every other day may be necessary to prevent recurrence.

Although corticosteroid therapy is usually the first-line treatment, other modalities are advocated. Anti-VEGF agents, such as topical (10 mg/mL) bevacizumab or subconjunctival (1.25 mg/0.05 mL) bevacizumab have shown promising results in corneal NV. Subconjunctival injections tend to be short lived and limited to active NV. Epitheliopathy and stromal thinning have been reported with long-term use of topical bevacizumab.[1] No current guidelines are available for optimal concentration and dosing regimen.

Occlusion of vessels with the use of argon laser photocoagulation and photodynamic therapy has been advocated as a treatment for corneal NV. Laser photocoagulation with 577 nm yellow dye has been used to obliterate vessels, but the vessels tend to reopen. Its use is limited in extensive corneal NV, and its role in stromal NV remains unclear.[2] Multiple applications may need to be performed for photodynamic therapy, and its high cost and potential systemic side effects may limit its use. Treatment should be tailored according to the needs of each patient. Topical corticosteroids are effective in the majority of cases if used properly. For persistent corneal stromal NV, other modalities are appropriate as adjunctive therapy as long-term efficacy and safety of other modalities have not been established.

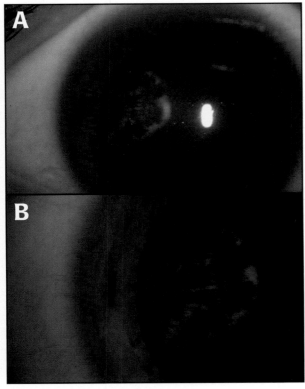

Figure 9-1. A 22-year-old patient with resolved contact lens-induced NV. Note the lipid keratopathy and regressed stromal NV (ghost vessels).

What if the Patient Wears Contact Lenses?

Both superficial and deep stromal NV can be seen with hydrogels (extended and daily-wear), hard (polymethyl methacrylate), and rigid gas-permeable (RGP) lenses (Figure 9-1).[3] For this patient with significant unilateral disease, herpetic keratitis is still on the top of my differential. It is possible that the deep stromal NV and diffuse stromal infiltrate is related to poor fitting or poor compliance, but I would expect the findings to be bilateral, although asymmetric. Slit-lamp exam with the current lens in place often reveals a tight fit. Contact lens-induced NV is more common in patients who are highly myopic, have ocular surface disease, or use extended-wear hydrogels. They should be refitted into daily wear, higher oxygen permeable silicone, or RGP lenses. Depending on the severity of the NV, contact lens wear may be contraindicated. Checking for corneal sensation, anterior chamber cell, and intraocular pressure can help differentiate contact lens-related NV from HSV keratitis.

References

1. Kim SW, Ha BJ, Kim EK, et al. The effect of topical bevacizumab on corneal neovascularization. *Ophthalmology.* 2008;115:e33-e38.
2. Primbs GB, Casey R, Wamser K, et al. Photodynamic therapy for corneal neovascularization. *Ophthalmic Surg Lasers.* 1998;29:832-838.
3. Foulks GN, Steffanson E, Hamilton RC. Regression of corneal neovascularization during silicone contact lens wear and the relationship to contact lens-induced anterior chamber hypoxia. *Cornea.* 1987;65:6-60.

SECTION II

EXTERNAL EYE DISEASE
AND TUMORS

How Should I Treat a Patient With Red Eye and Photophobia if My Exam Reveals Meibomian Gland Dysfunction and Foci of Subepithelial Infiltrates at the Limbus?

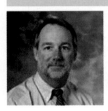

Neal P. Barney, MD

The presentation of staphylococcus marginal ulceration (staph marginal disease) includes unilateral sectoral redness, pain, and significant photophobia. These symptoms are preceded by a few days of worsening burning, irritation, or foreign body sensation. The most classically described findings are focal redness at the 2, 4, 8, or 10 o'clock limbus. The staph marginal ulcer is a 0.5- to 1.0-mm, grey-white, superficial, stromal infiltrate separated from the reddened limbus by a 1-mm clear zone of cornea (Figure 10-1). If multiple ulcers present, they are concentric with the limbus and may coalesce over time, giving a crescentric area of involvement. Initially, the epithelium overlying the infiltrate is intact but ulcerates over a few days.

Catarrhal ulcer is the term used historically to refer to marginal ulceration in general. Although an association with numerous different bacterial organisms is reported,[1] staphylococcus disease is most common for treatment considerations. The pathogenesis is considered to be secondary to the presence of considerable concentrations of bacterial cell products and not an active infection of the cornea. The source of staph bacterial products would be the periocular skin, lid margins, and conjunctiva. Another source may be blood-borne bacteria and their products circulating to the limbus. The limbus and peripheral cornea are highly immune reactive areas. The circulation at the limbus may predispose to immune complex deposition. Mast cell number is greater in the limbus than the rest of the conjunctiva. The peripheral cornea has greater concentrations of

Figure 10-1. Staphylococcal margin disease. The cornea has a grey-white, superficial, stromal infiltrate. Note the intervening clear area of cornea between the lesion and limbus.

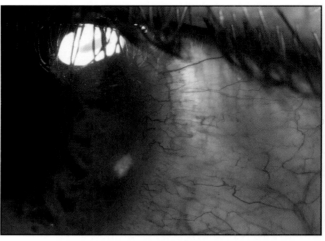

immunoglobulins and complement components than the central cornea. Finally, dendritic cells for antigen presentation are found normally in the epithelium of the peripheral cornea but not centrally.[2] A commonly proposed mechanism for staph marginal disease is the diffusion of bacterial products (antigens) into the peripheral cornea where they encounter antibody in a Gel and Coombs Type III hypersensitivity reaction. A polymorphonuclear cell infiltration ensues.

The differential diagnosis includes phlyctenule disease, peripheral ulcerative keratitis (PUK), Terrien's marginal degeneration, contact lens-associated microbial keratitis, Mooren's ulcer, sarcoidosis, and Thyseson's superficial punctate keratitis. Skin diseases such as rosacea and atopic dermatitis or eczema may predispose to staph marginal disease. Distinguishing characteristics of staph marginal disease are the presence of clear cornea between limbus and lesion, superficial stromal grey-white infiltrate, and lack of stromal loss. A phlyctenule will have a wedge-shaped leash of vessels, base at the limbus, and apex as a raised, grey-white, gelatinous-appearing lesion just onto the cornea.

The diagnosis is made based on the history and findings. The history should uncover any previous episodes, associated skin disease, contact lens use, or systemic disease. Exam should include careful inspection of the lids for collorettes (seborrhea), meibomian gland dysfunction (rosacea), or eczema (atopy). The conjunctiva should be examined for any lesions or nodules. Scleritis should be noted as it is often present with PUK. The corneal findings are those mentioned previously. There is seldom any anterior uveitis associated with staph marginal disease.

Initial Management

Treatment often brings significant relief of symptoms and signs rapidly. The use of antibiotic drops or ointment alone is recommended for any patient who is a contact lens wearer or who presents for the first time with staph marginal disease. Upon return in 3 to 4 days, the patient usually notes mild improvement. If no worsening is noted, a topical steroid (such as prednisolone acetate or phosphate 1% 4 times daily for 1 week) may be added while the antibiotics are continued. Often, the area involved appears as a faint, subepithelial scar with intact epithelium after this 1-week treatment. If so, the antibiotic and steroid may be stopped without taper. If the patient is not a contact lens wearer and is known to have previous episodes of staph marginal disease, then treatment may be initiated with a combination antibiotic-steroid drop such as tobramycin-dexamethasone or tobramycin-loteprednol etabonate 4 times per day. The patient should revisit in 1 week, and medications may be stopped if symptoms are improved and the lesion is resolved.

What if the Infiltrates Persist or Recur?

If the ulcer is not resolved after 1 week of combination therapy, consider a longer course of therapy. If there is stromal tissue loss, stop the treatment for 24 hours and perform a culture. If there is coalescence of a few adjacent ulcers, increase the frequency of the combination drops. The lid margin disease should be addressed as lid scrubs for seborrhea or rosacea. If meibomian gland dysfunction is significant, doxycycline 100 mg twice per day for 1 month then once per day for a month should be instituted. A systemic evaluation should be undertaken for any nonhealing ulcer or the presence of scleritis to include testing for sarcoid, rheumatoid arthritis, and Wegener's granulomatosis.

References

1. Duke-Elder S. *Diseases of the outer eye.* Vol VIII. London, UK: Kimpton; 1965.
2. Mondino BJ. Inflammatory diseases of the peripheral cornea. *Ophthalmology.* 1988;95:463-467.

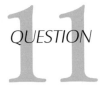

How Can I Help a 47-Year-old Female Who Uses Artificial Tears 6 Times Daily and Continues to Complain of Dry Eyes?

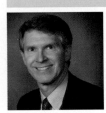

Stephen C. Pflugfelder, MD

The history suggests this patient has a chronic and severe dry eye condition. Evaluation should begin with a thorough systemic and ocular history with attention to symptoms of a systemic autoimmune condition, such as Sjögren's syndrome (SS) or rheumatoid arthritis. These would include symptoms of dry mouth; difficulty chewing and swallowing dry food; or painful, tender, or stiff joints. Currently taken systemic medications should be reviewed to identify any with anticholinergic effects that could be causing dry eye. Most commonly these include antihistamines, antispasmodics, and antidepressants. The patient should be questioned about the severity and nature of the ocular discomfort, with attention to exacerbating factors (eg, low humidity or computer use) and symptoms of blurred vision. The patient should be asked about the ability to reflex tear in response to emotional or environmental stimuli.

A detailed ocular surface and tear evaluation should be performed. The components of this exam should include visual acuity and evaluation of lid closure, blink rate, the presence of anterior or posterior blepharitis, and punctal position and patency. Conjunctival (scarring, chalasis, pinguecula, or pterygium) and corneal epithelial (punctate erosions, filaments, or epithelial defects) signs should be noted (Figure 11-1). If the patient is complaining of blurred vision, corneal topography should be performed to assess corneal smoothness. Irregularity or poor reflectivity of Placido rings or elevated surface regularity indices (eg, SRI) may be noted (Figure 11-2).[1] Fluorescein should be instilled using a fluorescein strip wet with preservative-free saline, and tear breakup time and presence,

Figure 11-1. Corneal topography showing marked irregularity of Placido rings and elevated surface regularity index (SRI).

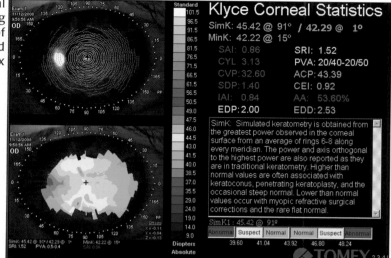

Figure 11-2. Corneal epithelial filaments stained with fluorescein.

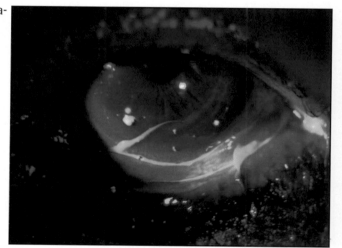

location, and severity of the corneal staining should be measured. Lissamine green staining to evaluate the conjunctiva should be performed, with attention to the exposure zone (Figure 11-3) and superior bulbar conjunctiva. Staining in the latter area is a sign of superior limbic keratoconjunctivitis. Tear production should be evaluated with a Schirmer test. In my hands, the Schirmer-I test performed without anesthesia provides the most valuable information because it tests ability to reflex tear in response to sensory stimulation. If the patient has a Schirmer test less than 5 mm and moderate-to-severe exposure zone corneal and conjunctival staining, I recommend the patient have serological testing to look for the presence of circulating autoantibodies associated with SS, including rheumatoid factor, antinuclear antibody, and SS-associated antibodies A and B. Consultation with a rheumatologist is suggested if autoantibodies are detected. Corneal sensitivity should be evaluated in selected cases, particularly when an exposure zone corneal epithelial defect is present.

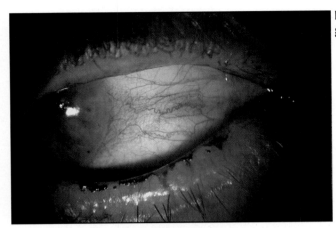

Figure 11-3. Conjunctival lissamine green staining in the exposure zone.

<u>Table 11-1</u>

Dry Eye Management

Treatment by Severity Level			
1	2	3	4
Education; environmental/dietary modification; elim. offending systemic medications; artificial tear substitutes, gels/ointments; lid therapy			→
	Anti-inflammatories; tetracyclines for meibomianitis, rosacea; plugs secretagogues; moisture chamber specs		→
		Serum; contact lenses; permanent punctal occlusion	→
			Systemic IS therapy; surgery (AMT lid surgery tarsorrhaphy, MM & SG transplant)

IS = immunosuppression; AMT = amniotic membrane transplant; MM = mucous membrane; SG = salivary gland

Treatment Options

My treatment regimen is based on the severity-based algorithm proposed by the Dry Eye WorkShop (DEWS) (Table 11-1).[2]

Generally, chronic dry eye that is not adequately treated with artificial tears will require one or more therapeutic agents. If tear production is 5 mm or less in the presence of moderate-to-severe ocular surface dye staining, punctal occlusion is performed.

Figure 11-4. Cornea with severe epitheliopathy and previous sterile ulcers fit with Boston Ocular Surface prosthesis, a sclera-bearing lens with a fluid-filled reservoir over the cornea.

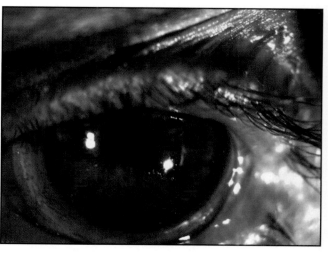

I recommend thermal cautery for patients who have lost the ability to reflex tear, while extended duration intracanalicular punctal plugs are used for patients who maintain the ability to reflex tear. Patients with reduced vision due to corneal epithelial disease require the most aggressive therapy, which typically would include preservative artificial tears, pulsed topical corticosteroid steroid (eg, loteprednol, etabonate 0.5% 4 times a day for 2 weeks followed by twice daily for 2 weeks), cyclosporine A 0.05% emulsion 2 to 4 times per day, oral doxycycline 40 mg per day (given in 1 or 2 doses), and topical autologous serum or plasma. If vision remains decreased or if the patient continues to complain of moderate-to-severe irritation or photophobia, the Boston Ocular Surface prosthesis is recommended (Figure 11-4).[3]

References

1. de Paiva CS, Lindsey JL, Pflugfelder SC. Assessing the severity of keratitis sicca with videokeratoscopic indices. *Ophthalmology*. 2003;110:1102-1109.
2. Management and Therapy Subcommittee of the International Dry Eye WorkShop. Management and therapy of dry eye disease: report of the Management and Therapy Subcommittee of the International Dry Eye WorkShop. *Ocul Surf*. 2007;5:163-178.
3. Romero-Rangel T, Stavrou P, Cotter J, Rosenthal P, Baltatzis S, Foster CS. Gas-permeable scleral contact lens therapy in ocular surface disease. *Am J Ophthalmol*. 2000;130:25-32.

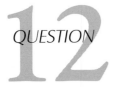

A 68-YEAR-OLD FEMALE WITH RHEUMATOID ARTHRITIS PRESENTS WITH A RED, PAINFUL EYE AND STROMAL MELT AT THE LIMBUS. HOW SHOULD I TREAT HER?

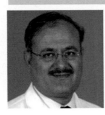

Virender S. Sangwan, MS

Peripheral ulcerative keratitis (PUK) is a crescent-shaped, destructive, inflammatory lesion of the perilimbal cornea associated with an epithelial defect and subepithelial cellular infiltrate at its advancing edge.[1,2] These features help differentiate PUK from non-inflammatory lesions such as Terrien's marginal degeneration (Figure 12-1). Most forms of PUK have associated inflammation of the adjacent conjunctiva, episclera, and sclera.

Roughly 50% of all cases of noninfectious PUK have an associated collagen vascular disease, with the most common being rheumatoid arthritis (RA) (Figure 12-1C) followed by Wegener's granulomatosis (WG) and infectious causes. Peripheral microbial keratitis (Figure 12-1D) progresses rapidly and usually responds to specific antibiotic therapy, while immunosuppressive therapy would be contraindicated in infectious PUK. Mooren's ulcer (Figure 12-1A), another form of PUK, is a painful, relentless, chronic ulcerative keratitis that begins peripherally and progresses centrally and circumferentially with complete absence of scleritis and diagnosable systemic disease. Absence of scleritis is of substantial clinical importance because many of the misdiagnosed cases of Mooren's ulcer had the PUK in association with adjacent scleritis, necrotizing or otherwise (Figure 12-1B). In Mooren's ulcer, there is involvement of limbus in contrast to PUK associated with RA and staphylococcal marginal disease where limbus is spared. PUK in different collagen vascular diseases does not have any specific presentation and features.

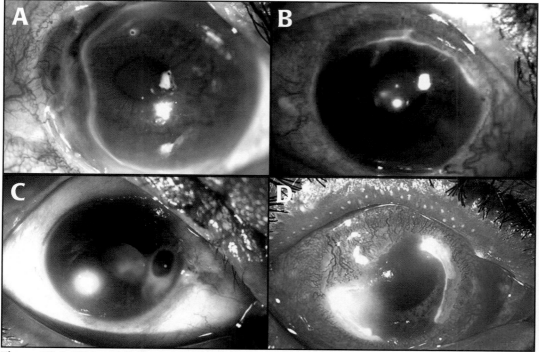

Figure 12-1. Slit-lamp photograph of a patient having typical features of Mooren's ulcer (A). Note the absence of associated scleritis and overhanging advancing edge with extreme thinning of ulcer bed. Slit-lamp photograph of a patient having peripheral keratopathy along with severe diffuse anterior scleritis (B). Slit-lamp photo of peripheral corneal perforation in a patient with RA (C). Note the absence of inflammation in the cornea adjacent to the perforation. Slit-lamp photo of peripheral infective keratitis with *Pseudomonas aeruginosa* (D). Note extensive slough-ing and discharge associated with ulceration as opposed to clean ulceration in patients with immune-mediated PUK.

PUK or keratopathy can be seen in patients with scleritis. This is a poor prognostic sign because scleritis patients with peripheral keratopathy more often have necrotizing scleri-tis (NS), decrease in vision, anterior uveitis, and impending corneal perforation. Presence of peripheral keratopathy and scleritis also indicates more likelihood of associated sys-temic disease.

Significance of Peripheral Ulcerative Keratitis in a Patient With Rheumatoid Arthritis

Development of NS or PUK in patients with RA carries a grim prognosis not only for the eye but also for life. It signifies that the destructive vasculitic process is present out-side joints to involve the sclera and potentially other extra-articular sites. These patients are at increased risk of death related to visceral vasculitic complications unless treated aggressively with systemic immunosuppressive agents.[3,4]

What Do You Watch for on Eye Examination?

RA patients with scleritis should be closely monitored for development of signs of NS and PUK. Red-free light examination should be done using the slit-lamp biomicroscopic examination to detect areas of cellular infiltration, ischemia, and vascular occlusion. Any peripheral keratopathy in these patients should be followed up closely and treated aggressively with appropriate topical and systemic therapy. Look for corneal involvement in every follow-up visit in patients with scleritis. Meticulous slit-lamp biomicroscopy should be performed to detect anterior uveitis or posterior segment disease. The clinician should collaborate with a rheumatologist to manage the involvement of other systems in such patients.

One should also be aware that surgical trauma may trigger inflammatory microangiopathy resulting in scleritis-associated PUK in patients with systemic vasculitis. It is crucial to identify susceptible patients prior to eye surgery in order to prevent postoperative ocular complications, which could be devastating to the eye and vision.

Systemic Work-Up

A thorough medical history and examination are mandatory, as is comprehensive laboratory investigation. The purpose of workup is to rule out the presence of an occult systemic disease unless diagnosed already; to assess the extent of systemic visceral involvement, if any; and to establish baseline clinical and laboratory data so that treatment-induced side effects can be monitored. The investigation should include complete blood cell counts with differential, rheumatoid factor, antinuclear antibody assay, circulating immune complexes, liver function tests, venereal disease research laboratory test and fluorescent treponemal antibody absorption test, blood urea nitrogen and creatinine, urinalysis, and a chest X-ray or computed tomography. Additional testing might be indicated by review of systems and physical examination.

Treatment

A patient presenting with PUK and RA represents a true ophthalmic emergency, because this is a potentially life- and sight-threatening condition that can progress rapidly. Therefore, communication and prompt referral to a rheumatologist comfortable with cytotoxic immunosuppressive agents for initiation of therapy is of utmost importance. If the treating ophthalmologist is trained in prescribing and monitoring this type of treatment, then referral to a rheumatologist may not be necessary. Current recommended treatment is systemic corticosteroids in combination with an immunosuppressive agent. Although higher doses of corticosteroids are typically needed initially to achieve rapid control of inflammation, the long-term goal is to control the inflammation with an immunosuppressive drug that is capable of reducing the dose of corticosteroids to none or minimal. These medications not only can improve the activity of systemic disease and ocular inflammation, but can also improve the corneal graft survival in patients with RA.

After ruling out an infectious cause of PUK, intense topical steroid therapy should be initiated (eg, hourly prednisolone acetate 1% eyedrops), and conjunctival resection with tissue adhesive and bandage contact lens application should be done at the earliest. Prophylactic antibiotic eyedrops and a cycloplegic agent should also be started. Conjunctival resection may reduce access of leukocytes and other immune mediators to the peripheral cornea, resulting in decreased release of collagenases and proteinases and subsequent stromal melt. Tissue adhesives create an effective barrier to leukocytes from tear film to cornea, further preventing stromal melt. Because patients with PUK and RA have associated keratoconjunctivitis sicca, it is imperative that frequent lubrication should also be started. Punctal occlusion should be considered in selected cases.

Surgical management should be reserved for PUK patients with corneal perforation or thinning that threatens structural integrity of the eye. A concomitant effective immunosuppressive therapy is critical for controlling immune-mediated inflammation and preventing graft melt. Options include penetrating keratoplasty, lamellar keratoplasty, or patch graft depending on the extent of involvement. In the presence of severe dry eye, tarsorrhaphy may enhance the chance of graft survival. The visual outcome after penetrating keratoplasty or patch graft in this patient population remains poor.

References

1. Messemer EM, Foster CS. Vasculitic peripheral ulcerative keratitis. *Surv Ophthalmol.* 1999;43:379-396.
2. Ladas JG, Mondino BJ. Systemic disorders associated with peripheral corneal ulceration. *Curr Opin Ophthalmol.* 2000;11:468-471.
3. Sangwan VS, Panayotis Z, Foster CS. Mooren's ulcer: current concepts in diagnosis and management. *Ind J Ophthalmol.* 1997;45(1):7-17.
4. Foster CS, Forstot SL, Wilson LA. Mortality rate in rheumatoid arthritis patients developing necrotizing scleritis or peripheral ulcerative keratitis. Effects of immunosuppression. *Ophthalmology.* 1984;91:1253-1263.

A 47-Year-Old Hispanic Male Complains of a "Growth" in the Corner of His Right Eye. Does His Pterygium Need to Be Removed?

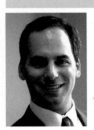

William Trattler, MD

Pterygia are elevated fibrovascular lesions on the surface of the eye that arise from the conjunctiva and extend onto the corneal surface. Pterygia most commonly appear nasally. As they grow, they can induce astigmatism and can eventually grow into the visual axis. Pterygia are more common in areas of the world with higher levels of ultraviolet light exposure.

Examination and Medical Management

When patients present with pterygia, I find that it is important to determine the location of the pterygium as well as the extent to which the pterygium encroaches onto the cornea (Figure 13-1). Is the pterygium encroaching on the visual axis? How much astigmatism has been induced? Is there any loss of best-corrected vision? Just as important, I also carefully inspect the pterygium to make sure that we are not dealing with carcinoma in situ or squamous cell carcinoma. I also perform a corneal topography to assess the degree that the shape of the cornea is influenced by the pterygium, as well as take a photo to document the size and location of the lesion.

For many patients, their main complaint with small pterygia is ocular redness. In my experience, I have been successful at improving the cosmetic appearance of small pterygia by addressing the ocular surface. Patients are placed on a course of topical

Figure 13-1. Primary pterygium encroaching on visual axis and inducing some corneal astigmatism

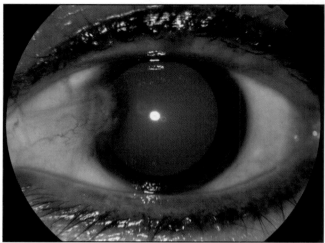

steroids, lubricating drops and gels, along with topical cyclosporine. Some patients with significant dry eye may benefit from punctal plugs. Over 4 to 6 weeks, patients typically notice an improvement in the degree of conjunctival hyperemia, and often surgery can be avoided.

Surgical Management

When the pterygium grows onto the cornea and encroaches into the visual axis, surgical intervention is required. I advise patients that, even with a perfect surgery, there is a possibility of reduced uncorrected and/or best-corrected visual acuity, and the amount of astigmatism present can increase or decrease. There is, of course, also a risk of pterygium recurrence. As well, there can be cosmetic changes to the eye that can last for many months, such as low-grade conjunctival redness.

There are numerous techniques for pterygium excision that have been designed to reduce the risk of recurrence as well as improve the postoperative cosmetic appearance.

With pterygium surgery, there are a few decision points:

1. Whether to use mitomycin C (MMC) to reduce the risk of recurrence

2. Whether to use a graft (amniotic vs conjunctival autograft)

3. Whether to use fibrin glue versus sutures to secure the flap

Mitomycin C

Although MMC is very effective at preventing recurrence of pterygium, the major concern with using MMC is a scleral melt. The most important teaching points to avoid a scleral melt include avoiding excessive scleral cautery and avoiding exposure of MMC directly to the scleral bed. Additionally, following surgery, it is critical to lubricate the eye, as dry eye can also lead to a scleral melt.

There are a number of methods for using MMC to reduce the risk of pterygium recurrence. The most popular is to soak pieces of a Murocel sponge in MMC, and then take these sponges and apply them directly to the subconjunctival tissue for 2 to 5 minutes. An alternative treatment strategy was developed by Alfred Anduze of the US Virgin Islands.[1] At the conclusion of the pterygium excision, he recommends injection of 0.1 mL of 0.2 mg/mL (0.02%) into the subconjunctival tissue. Some surgeons in the past have recommended MMC eyedrops for a few weeks to months postoperatively, but the risk of a serious complication has dramatically reduced the popularity of this technique.[2]

Following either MMC application technique, the eye should be rinsed with balanced salt solution. These MMC application techniques can be used with amniotic grafts, primary closure with sutures, and even the bare sclera technique.

Other techniques of MMC usage include subconjunctival injections prior to surgery to potentially reduce the size of the pterygium as well as injection of MMC postoperatively if there are early signs of recurrence.[3]

In my practice, I have adopted the Anduze technique of MMC usage. Over 5 years, this technique appears both safe and effective for my patients.

GRAFT VERSUS NO GRAFT

Decades of research has determined that applying a graft over the bare sclera can reduce the risk of recurrence. Numerous studies have looked at both conjunctival autografts and amniotic membrane grafts. Both techniques are very effective at reducing the risk of recurrence. Some studies have suggested that the conjunctival autograft is the superior technique.[4] However, the difference between an autograft and an amniotic graft are small, especially when MMC is also applied. Amniotic grafts are also extremely simple to use, as they arrive at the surgery center prepared and ready for use.

In cases where the pterygium is present both nasally and temporally, amniotic grafts are the preferred method for covering the scleral bed compared to conjunctival autografts. This is because the removal of both the nasal and temporal pterygia will leave a very large conjunctival defect. Thankfully, amniotic membrane grafts come in various sizes, and one can easily order a size that can be used to cover both sides.

SUTURES VERSUS FIBRIN GLUE

For numerous years, grafts have been secured in place with sutures. Nylon suture works very well, but because they do not dissolve, they have to be removed during the postoperative period. An absorbable suture material such as polyglactin 9-0 (Vicryl) can be used as an alternative. However, Vicryl tends to induce more inflammation than nylon and may therefore increase the likelihood of pterygium recurrence.[5,6]

Fibrin glue has been used for the past 5 to 7 years during pterygium surgery. It is a simple and straightforward method for securing either conjunctival autografts or amniotic membrane grafts. The use of glue reduces surgical time, although it is more costly than sutures. Another potential disadvantage of using fibrin glue is possible dislodging of the graft edge or even the entire graft during the postoperative period. Some surgeons advocate placing 4 cardinal sutures along with fibrin glue to prevent this complication.

My Preferences

The choice of treatment of pterygium varies between geographical regions and between surgeons. I practice in South Florida, an area with high ultraviolet light intensity, and I treat all of my cases virtually the same, whether they are primary or recurrent. I apply MMC at the time of pterygium excision in each patient. I prefer the Anduze technique (ie, injecting 0.1 mL or less of MMC into the subconjunctival tissue at the end of the procedure). I prefer amniotic membrane graft over conjunctival autografts. One important factor that is critical for reducing the recurrence of pterygium is to aggressively suppress inflammation following surgery. Kheirkhah et al showed that inflammation can be a major factor in pterygium recurrence.[7] I have switched to the use of stronger topical corticosteroids such as difluprednate during the initial 4 to 6 weeks after surgery, and I also extended the use of topical steroids in my patients to 8 to 10 weeks postoperatively.

Another important factor to identify and treat is dry eye. It is common for the eye to develop dryness after pterygium excision, which can, in some cases, lead to dellen formation and scleral melts. Dry eye is even more common when both nasal and temporal pterygia are removed at the same setting. I, therefore, often place punctal plugs to raise the tear film, and I prescribe topical cyclosporine to reduce inflammation and improve the quality of tears. Multiple studies in the peer-reviewed literature have reported a reduced risk of pterygium recurrence when topical cyclosporine is used postoperatively.[8]

References

1. Anduze AL. Pterygium surgery with mitomycin-C: ten-year results. *Ophthalmic Surg Lasers.* 2001;32(4):341-345.
2. Singh G, Wilson MR, Foster CS. Long-term follow-up study of mitomycin eyedrops as adjunctive treatment of pterygia and its comparison with conjunctival autograft transplantation. *Cornea.* 1990;9(4):331-334.
3. Donnenfeld ED, Perry HD, Fromer S, Doshi S, Solomon R, Biser S. Subconjunctival mitomycin C as adjunctive therapy before pterygium excision. *Ophthalmology.* 2003;110(5):1012-1016.
4. Oguz H. Amniotic membrane grafting versus conjunctival autografting in pterygium surgery. *Clin Experiment Ophthalmol.* 2005;33(4):447-448.
5. Bahar I, Weinberger D, Gaton DD, Avisar R. Fibrin glue versus vicryl sutures for primary conjunctival closure in pterygium surgery: long-term results. *Curr Eye Res.* 2007;32(5):399-405.
6. Uy HS, Reyes JM, Flores JD, Lim-Bon-Siong R. Comparison of fibrin glue and sutures for attaching conjunctival autografts after pterygium excision. *Ophthalmology.* 2005;112(4):667-671.
7. Kheirkhah A, Casas V, Sheha H, Raju VK, Tseng SC. Role of conjunctival inflammation in surgical outcome after amniotic membrane transplantation with or without fibrin glue for pterygium. *Cornea.* 2008;27(1):56-63.
8. Ibáñez M, Eugarrios MF, Calderón DI. Topical cyclosporin A and mitomycin C injection as adjunctive therapy for prevention of primary pterygium recurrence. *Ophthalmic Surg Lasers Imaging.* 2009;40(3):239-244.

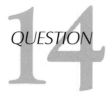

A Patient Diagnosed With Bell's Palsy 2 Days Ago Presents With Lagophthalmos and Moderate Superficial Punctate Keratopathy Inferiorly on the Cornea. How Should I Treat Her?

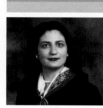

Natalie A. Afshari, MD, FACS
(co-authored with Brad H. Feldman, MD)

Bell's palsy is a peripheral facial nerve paralysis that evolves over hours to days and occurs in the absence of central nervous system disease. It is almost universally unilateral (99.7%), rarely recurrent (<10%), and typically transient, with nearly all patients improving over time. Remission usually occurs within 4 weeks of the onset of paralysis. However, delayed improvement can be seen for up to 6 months, and up to 17% have some degree of permanent paralysis. It is more common in pregnant women, in patients with diabetes mellitus, and in those with a positive family history.[1] While considered a diagnosis of exclusion, it accounts for approximately two-thirds of acute facial palsies and is often characterized by a constellation of recognizable symptoms beyond seventh nerve involvement (Table 14-1).[2]

Reactivation of herpes simplex virus is now generally thought to be responsible for Bell's palsy. The facial nerve may be particularly susceptible to injury from inflammation because of mechanical compression within the narrow meatal foramen in the temporal bone. Oral prednisone and acyclovir are often given to Bell's palsy patients early in the disease (ideally, within 72 hours) in attempts to mitigate the disease course.[3] There is no consensus on the effect of these treatments, but the potential benefits and minimal risks support a 10-day course of oral prednisone (60 mg taper) and acyclovir (400 mg 5 times a day).

Table 14-1
Constellation of Symptoms of Bell's Palsy

Incidence	Symptom
100%	Facial nerve paralysis
80%	Hypersensitivity of face to temperature, wind and touch
60%	Ear pain
57%	Alterations in taste (dysgeusia)
30%	Decreased tolerance to everyday sounds (hyperacusis)
17%	Decreased tearing

Adapted from Adour KK. Current concepts in neurology diagnosis and management of facial paralysis. *N Engl J Med.* 1982;307:348-351.

Evaluation

Care must be taken to examine the external ear, auditory canal, and tympanic membrane for the vesicles that are typical of Ramsay Hunt syndrome from herpes zoster, an entity with a poorer prognosis of facial nerve recovery. An audiogram is also important to rule out asymmetric hearing loss from vestibulocochlear involvement. Whenever there is evidence of multiple cranial nerve, bilateral, atypical, or central nervous system involvement, a workup must begin to rule out neoplastic, inflammatory, or autoimmune etiologies. In these cases, magnetic resonance imaging with gadolinium is recommended, as is consultation with an ear, nose, and throat or neurology specialist.

Beyond the disfigurement of the Bell's facial droop, the primary concern for these patients is ocular secondary to dysfunctional blinking, a widened palpebral fissure, and poor eyelid closure due to a deinnervated orbicularis oculi and the unopposed eyelid retractors (Figure 14-1). The severity of facial nerve paralysis and lid closure is graded with the House-Brackmann criteria (Table 14-2).[4] Exposure keratopathy from poor lid closure is further exacerbated by a degraded tear film due to increased evaporation; inadequate tear replenishment; disrupted mixing of the mucin, lipid, and aqueous components; and, occasionally, decreased tear production.

Management

The management of exposure keratopathy begins with frequent preservative-free artificial tears throughout the day and more viscous gels or ointments at bedtime. Nocturnal lagophthalmos is addressed most effectively with eyelid taping or placement of a cellophane dressing over the eye to retain moisture. Some patients may benefit from moisture chamber glasses or goggles, and others will require frequent applications of daytime gels or ointments. Slit-lamp examination of these patients typically reveals inferior punctate

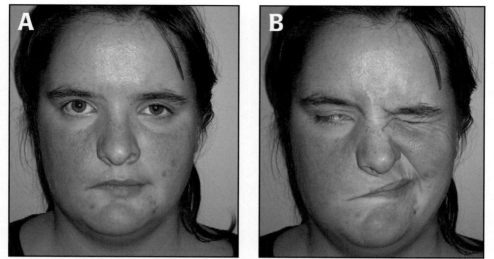

Figure 14-1. Right facial droop, nasolabial flattening, and widened palpebral fissure (A). Residual lagophthalmos despite forceful eyelid closure (B). (Reprinted with permission from Kumar A, Ryzenman J, Barr A. Revision facial nerve surgery. *Otolaryngol Clin North Am.* 2006;39(4):815-832.)

<u>Table 14-2</u>

House-Brackmann Grading System for Facial Paralysis

Grade	Definition
I	Normal symmetrical function in all areas
II	Slight weakness noticeable only on close inspection Complete eye closure with minimal effort Slight asymmetry of smile with maximal effort Synkinesis barely noticeable, contracture, or spasm absent
III	Obvious weakness, but not disfiguring May not be able to lift eyebrow Complete eye closure and strong but asymmetrical mouth movement with maximal effort Obvious but not disfiguring synkinesis, mass movement, or spasm
IV	Obvious disfiguring weakness Inability to lift brow Incomplete eye closure and asymmetry of mouth with maximal effort Severe synkinesis, mass movement, spasm
V	Motion barely perceptible Incomplete eye closure, slight movement corner mouth Synkinesis, contracture, and spasm usually absent
VI	No movement Loss of tone No synkinesis, contracture, or spasm

Adapted from House JW, Brackmann DE. Facial nerve grading system. *Otolaryngol Head Neck Surg.* 1985;93:146-147.

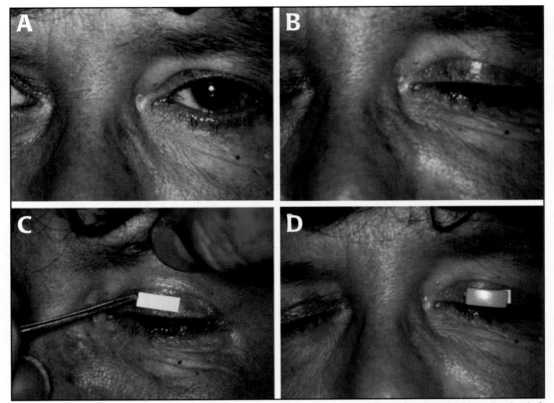

Figure 14-2. Application of lid weight for lagophthalmos. Uncorrected lagophthalmos in the left eye due to Bell's palsy with inferior and lateral injection due to exposure (A). 3mm of lagophthalmos on forced closure (B). Application of temporary upper lid weight (C). Resolution of lagophthalmos with lid weight (D). (Reprinted with permission from Rahman I, Sadiq SA. Ophthalmic management of facial nerve palsy: a review. *Surv Ophthalmol.* 2007;52(2):121-144.)

keratopathy, but this location may vary depending on the degree of nocturnal globe elevation (Bell's phenomenon). Note that in-office testing of Bell's phenomenon does not correlate well with nocturnal globe positioning and is of limited prognostic value.

All patients, including those with only mild exposure keratopathy on initial consultation, are generally seen within a week to assess progression. For patients demonstrating persistent moderate to severe exposure keratopathy, aggressive measures including tarsorrhaphy or gold weight placement are warranted to avoid corneal scarring, ulceration, or infection. Gold weights provide for gravitational closure of the upper eyelid, hold a considerable cosmetic advantage over tarsorrhaphy, and do not delay recovery of orbicularis function even when employed early in the course of disease. In order to optimize lid positioning, gold weights of 0.6 to 1.8 g can be trialed externally with tape before pretarsal implantation (Figure 14-2). Ninety percent of patients improve with gold weights, even though many have some residual lagophthalmos. Patients must be instructed to elevate their heads at night, and possible complications include migration or extrusion of the implant, as well as associated inflammation.[3]

In severe cases that progress to corneal ulceration, suture tarsorrhaphy is required to ensure adequate corneal coverage and avoid further melting or secondary infection.

Following resolution of ulceration, the tarsorrhaphy can be cautiously opened and re-evaluated. At this point, the lagophthalmos may be treated with a combination of lid tightening, loading, and reanimation procedures tailored to the individual. In selected cases of moderate to severe exposure keratopathy, botulinum toxin injection into Müller's muscle and levator can be attempted to achieve an upper lid ptosis lasting several weeks, but this effect typically takes 4 to 5 days, leads to variable degrees of coverage, and produces a poor cosmetic result. The main advantage is that, once the induced ptosis resolves, most patients will have had adequate spontaneous recovery of orbicularis function to necessitate no further intervention.

Infrequently, there is a role for high water content hydrogel contact lenses or rigid gas-permeable scleral lenses in combination with the frequent use of preservative-free artificial tears to both supplement the tear reservoir and enhance visual acuity through the artificial smooth refractive surface. When using therapeutic contact lenses, we prescribe topical fluoroquinolones for bacterial prophylaxis.

References

1. Mattox DE. Clinical disorders of the facial nerve. In Cummings CW, Flint PW, Harker LA, et al. *Cummings Otolaryngology: Head and Neck Surgery.* 4th ed. St. Louis, MO: Mosby; 2005:3333-3340.
2. Adour KK. Current concepts in neurology diagnosis and management of facial paralysis. *N Engl J Med.* 1982;307:348-351.
3. Rahman I, Sadiq SA. Ophthalmic management of facial nerve palsy: a review. *Surv Ophthalmol.* 2007;52: 121-144.
4. House JW, Brackmann DE. Facial nerve grading system. *Otolaryngol Head Neck Surg.* 1985;93:146-147.

A 43-Year-Old Female Is Complaining of Dry Eyes. The Exam Shows Punctate Keratopathy in the Inferior Third of Her Corneas. What Is the Optimal Management?

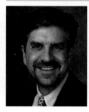

Jeffrey P. Gilbard, MD

Dry Eye Versus Meibomitis

Because the symptoms of dry eye are very similar to the symptoms of meibomitis and because both can cause punctate keratopathy in the inferior third of the cornea, the first step is to determine the basis for this patient's "dry eye" symptoms. Patients with dry eye complain of sandy-gritty irritation, burning, or, in early disease, an increased "awareness" of their eyes that gets worse as the day goes on. That is because elevated tear film osmolarity causes dry eye symptoms, and eye closure at night forms a watertight seal, blocking tear film evaporation, lowering elevated tear film osmolarity, and permitting the ocular surface a chance to recover. On eye opening, evaporation begins, tear film osmolarity increases as the day goes on,[1] and symptoms get worse as the day goes on. In contrast, patients with meibomitis complain of sandy-gritty irritation or burning, with or without eye redness, which is worse upon eye opening. This is because eye closure at night brings the inflamed eyelids up against the cornea, releasing inflammatory cytokines that have all night to irritate the cornea and inflame the ocular surface. With eye opening, tear flow increases, and symptoms improve quickly, even before breakfast. As meibomitis progresses, these patients develop meibomian gland dysfunction with deficiency of the tear film lipid layer, increased tear film evaporation, increased tear film osmolarity, and a second symptom peak toward the end of the day. As the eyelid inflammation burns out, the morning symptoms resolve, and the patient is left with a single symptom peak at the end of the day.[2]

Both dry eye and meibomitis can cause punctate keratopathy of the inferior third of the cornea. The 2 conditions can be differentiated by the pattern of diurnal variation, the tear film quality and quantity, and the pattern of surface staining. The best way to examine the tear film is to take a fluorescein strip, wet it with sterile saline, shake off the excess, and then pull the lower lid down and paint the strip across the inferior tarsal conjunctiva and have the patient blink. Examine the tear film with the cobalt blue light. In mild dry eye, the tear film will fluoresce and look normal. The first sign of decreased tear secretion will be absence of fluorescence in the nasal portion of the inferior marginal tear strip. As tear secretion drops further, the tear film will not fluoresce, then as secretion drops further, the tear film will look more "viscous"—the tear film, rather than snapping up as the upper lid rises after a blink, will move more slowly. Then, debris will appear in the pre-ocular tear film, and, finally, as secretion decreases further, a dehydrated mucous strand will appear in the inferior fornix. In pure dry eye, the conjunctiva will stain more than the cornea, and the nasal conjunctiva will stain more than the temporal conjunctiva (Figure 15-1). With careful observation, this staining can be seen with fluorescein, lissamine green, or rose bengal. Because fluorescein dye is already in the eye, I rarely find it necessary to add lissamine green or rose bengal, although patterns can be more easily seen with these dyes. Lissamine green is more comfortable for the patient than rose bengal.

In patients with meibomitis, patients with meibomitis/meibomian gland dysfunction, and those with both, the tear film fluoresces (Figure 15-2). As meibomian gland dysfunction increases, the tear film appears more watery in quality. The oil layer lowers the surface tension of the tear film, and, as this oil layer is lost, the tear film takes on this watery appearance. Most patients with mild meibomitis usually have no surface staining. At first, there will be staining of the inferior bulbar and/or superior bulbar conjunctiva under where the lid sits all day. But as the inflammation increases, the cornea stains at least as much as the conjunctiva.

Management

I would start the patient with dry eye on hypotonic tear-film electrolyte-matched preservative-free TheraTears 4 times daily with saturation dosing aiming to normalize elevated tear film osmolarity as quickly as possible. Saturation dosing involves splitting the content of a single-use container between both eyes in a sequential manner. Each drop osmotically rehydrates the osmotically dehydrated ocular surface. At the same time, I would start dietary supplementation with TheraTears Nutrition with flaxseed oil that improves the oil layer and fish oil that suppresses inflammation. Warm compresses also thicken the oil layer, reduce tear film evaporation, and have been shown to decrease surface staining, improve tear film break-up time, and improve dry eye symptoms.[3] These are particularly helpful if performed in the early afternoon, prior to the symptom peak that occurs in the afternoon. So, I would recommend an early afternoon warm compress for 2 to 5 minutes. Patients may find it helpful to use the iHeat Portable Warm Compress System (Advanced Vision Research, Woburn, MA) that maintains an evidence-based temperature of 105°F for 5 minutes.[4]

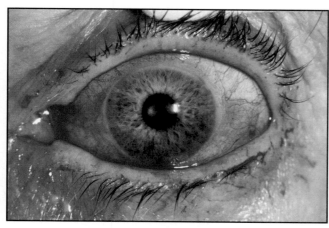

Figure 15-1. In pure dry eye, the conjunctiva will stain more than the cornea, and the nasal conjunctiva will stain more than the temporal conjunctiva.

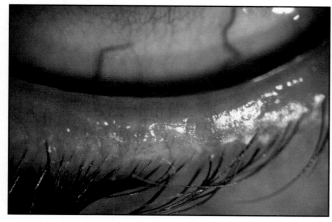

Figure 15-2. This patient with meibomitis has clean lashes, sharp margins, telangiectatic blood vessels crossing the lid margin, and stenosis of the meibomian gland orifices (orifices that are not visible but from which oil can be expressed).

Patients with meibomitis are started on doxycycline 50 to 100 mg a day to suppress inflammation and address the bacterial overgrowth[5] that causes the meibomian gland inflammation, TheraTears Nutrition to thin the meibomian gland oils and further suppress meibomian gland inflammation, and warm compress to thin meibomian gland oils and improve meibomian gland oil flow. The NutriDox Kit (Advanced Vision Research) provides 75 mg a day of doxycycline, TheraTears Nutrition, and the iHeat Portable Warm Compress System in a convenient treatment kit. After symptom improvement, I would manage the patient on TheraTears Nutrition, warm compress, and substitute doxycycline with SteriLid (Advanced Vision Research) to control the tendency these patients have for bacterial overgrowth.

References

1. Farris RL, Stuchell RN, Mandel ID. Tear osmolarity variation in the dry eye. *Trans Am Ophthalmol Soc.* 1986;84:250-268.
2. Gilbard JP. Human tear film electrolyte concentrations in health and dry-eye disease. *Int Ophthalmol Clin.* 1994;34(1):27-36.

3. Goto E, Monden Y, Takano Y, et al. Treatment of non-inflamed obstructive meibomian gland dysfunction by an infrared warm compression device. *Br J Ophthalmol.* 2002;86(12):1403-1407.
4. Olson MC, Korb DR, Greiner JV. Increase in tear film lipid layer thickness following treatment with warm compresses in patients with meibomian gland dysfunction. *Eye Contact Lens.* 2003;29(2):96-99.
5. Groden LR, Murphy B, Rodnite J, et al. Lid flora in blepharitis. *Cornea.* 1991;10(1):50-53.

Dr. Jeff Gilbard wrote an excellent chapter on dry eyes and meibomitis. Jeff died in an accident shortly after writing this chapter, and his contributions to ophthalmology will be missed. Jeff had a passion for the treatment of dry eyes and associated conditions, so much so that he formed his own company and was continually coming up with new treatments to help those with dry eyes. Jeff's chapter is heavily referenced with his own products, but each of his products sprung from his unique and detailed persistence in finding the causes and treatments for dry eyes.
—*Francis W. Price, Jr. MD*

A 42-Year-Old Female With Sectoral Redness in Her Right Eye Complains of Irritation in One Eye, but No Pain. How Should I Treat Her Episcleritis?

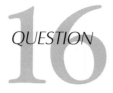

Albert S. Jun, MD, PhD

A red eye can present as a challenge. As in any case, the history is the first step to diagnosis. Consider the following questions:

* Is this the first time the eye has been red?
* How long has it been red?
* Have you been exposed to any irritants?
* Do you wear contacts?
* Do you have any tearing?
* Is the eye painful?
* How is your general health?

Of utmost importance is to rule out vision-threatening etiologies first. At this point, you may have episcleritis and scleritis left on your differential diagnosis. Here, a careful clinical examination helps with the diagnosis.

Episcleritis Versus Scleritis—Key Clinical Features

A key historical feature of scleritis is significant pain, typically worse with palpation through the lids or with moving the areas of overlying, hyperemic, and/or edematous conjunctiva. The pain often is characterized as dull or pressure like and can be severe enough to awaken a patient from sleep. Severe pain is not typical of episcleritis, but nearly half will complain of a discomfort such as a foreign body sensation.

A key examination finding in scleritis is a violaceous hue appearing deeper than the superficial radial redness of episcleritis. Use of a topical vasoconstrictor can be helpful, as it will blanch episcleritis. The vasoconstrictor, typically 2.5% phenylephrine, can be applied on a cotton-tipped applicator over the area of hyperemia or simply by instilling the drops on the ocular surface and observing for any changes in 5 to 10 minutes. Finally, typically, half of all scleritis cases are bilateral, whereas only one-third of all episcleritis cases are bilateral.[1]

Anatomy and Morphology

The episcleral space lies above the sclera and below the Tenon's capsule and contains loose, well-vascularized, connective tissue. Episcleritis is divided into 2 categories: simple and nodular. In simple episcleritis, uniform radial redness of the episclera is visible, either within a sector (Figure 16-1) or extending diffusely from the limbus, past the area of conjunctiva exposed in the interpalpebral fissure (Figure 16-2). In nodular episcleritis, vascular congestion is present with the addition of a discrete mobile elevation within the episcleral space.

Etiology

Episcleritis is often correctly labeled as idiopathic; however, one-third of cases have an underlying systemic association. Such diseases include atopy, gout, and vasculitic auto-immune diseases such as rheumatoid arthritis, systemic lupus erythematosus, relapsing polychondritis, and Wegener's granulomatosis. Other common conditions include serone-gative arthritic conditions, including inflammatory bowel disease and psoriasis. Infectious etiologies including syphilis and herpes simplex virus should also be considered.[2]

Management

The number of occurrences is an important consideration for treatment. Patients who present with their first episode typically are treated with artificial tears, as idiopathic etiology is the most common and has a self-limited course. All patients presenting with episcleritis should have an extensive review of systems. Patients with a positive review of systems may warrant laboratory investigation while starting treatment with topical lubrication. The initial set of tests can include a complete blood count (CBC), serum uric acid, antinuclear antibody (ANA), rheumatoid factor, erythrocyte sedimentation rate (ESR),

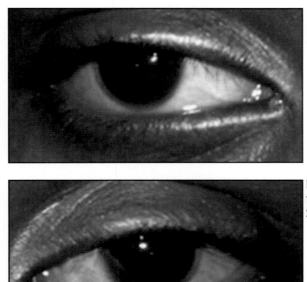

Figure 16-1. Simple episcleritis with temporal sector involvement. (Photo courtesy of Shameema Sikder, MD.)

Figure 16-2. Simple episcleritis with diffuse involvement. (Photo courtesy of Shameema Sikder, MD.)

venereal disease research laboratory (VDRL) test, fluorescent treponemal antibody absorption (FTA-ABS) test, and chest X-ray.[1,3] These tests can be undertaken with the help of the patient's primary care physician.

In recurrent cases or cases that fail to improve on topical lubrication, more aggressive treatment can be used. A low-potency steroid, such as fluorometholone 1% eye drops, 4 times a day is often used. Failure on this treatment can prompt an increase in frequency or a change to prednisolone acetate 1% eye drops 4 times a day. The next step would include using an oral nonsteroidal anti-inflammatory drug (NSAID), such as indomethacin 25 mg 3 times a day. Patients who do not respond to one NSAID may respond to another. It is important to note intraocular pressures before treatment with steroids of any type and duration, as intraocular pressure increases are possible. Furthermore, a stomach ulcer prophylactic medicine, such as ranitidine or omeprazole, should be prescribed with oral NSAIDs.[3]

Episcleritis affects men and women, both young and middle-aged, and usually resolves within 21 days. Typically, we ask patients to return for follow-up in 3 to 4 weeks if placed on topical lubrication and within 2 weeks if placed on steroids. As the episodes of episcleritis are self-limiting, topical lubrication can be continued as needed, and topical steroids can quickly be tapered. In cases where episcleritis becomes chronic or recurrent with a negative workup, a biopsy should be considered. Having the patient use topical steroids on an as-needed basis can lead to poor follow-up with sequelae such as increased intraocular pressure and cataract formation and is not recommended. Episcleritis is often idiopathic and resolves with minimal intervention; however, an effort should be made to understand its underlying etiology, especially in cases of recurrence.

Acknowledgment: The author thanks Shameema Sikder, MD, for assistance with manuscript preparation.

References

1. Watson PG, Hayreh SS. Scleritis and episcleritis. *Br J Ophthalmol.* 1976;60:163-191.
2. Akpek EK, Uy HS, Christen W, et al. Severity of episcleritis and systemic disease association. *Ophthalmology.* 1999;106:729-731.
3. Jabs DA, Mudun A, Dunn JP, et al. Episcleritis and scleritis: clinical features and treatment results. *Am J Ophthalmol.* 2000;130:469-476.

A 53-Year-Old Female Came to My Office With Sectoral Redness and Pain in One Eye. How Should I Manage Her Scleritis?

Sana S. Siddique, MD
(co-authored with C. Stephen Foster, MD, FACR, FACS)

Scleritis is a condition that may range from a benign, self-limited, superficial inflammation to a deeper, destructive involvement of the sclera. It is imperative to differentiate between scleritis and episcleritis because the former is not only associated with underlying systemic disorders, ocular morbidity, and mortality, but the treatment modalities differ vastly.

Signs and symptoms of scleritis include pain, globe tenderness to palpation, and ocular redness. The pain is often so intense as to wake the patient from sleep and tends to radiate to the forehead, jaw, temple, and sinuses.

The redness associated with scleritis usually has a bluish/violaceous tinge with injection of the deep episcleral blood vessels. It may be localized or diffuse and may occur simultaneously in both eyes.

Peripheral keratopathy in a patient with scleritis is an ominous ocular sign because such patients more often evolve to have necrotizing scleritis and impending corneal perforation.[1]

The classification scheme of Watson and Hayreh[2] and of Foster and Sainz de la Maza[1] has divided scleral disorders into scleritis and episcleritis (Figure 17-1).

Posterior scleritis is characterized by flattening of the posterior globe and thickening of the retinochoroid layer. Posterior scleritis is suspected when patients present with pain, worsened with eye movement, and visualization of serous retinal detachment, swollen optic nerve head, or circumscribed fundus mass. The diagnosis of posterior scleritis can be confirmed with ultrasonographic demonstration of the signs described above.

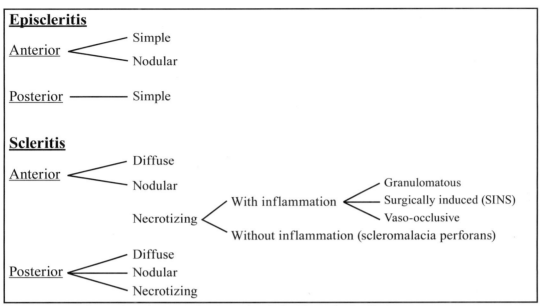

Figure 17-1. Schematic subcategorization of episcleritis and scleritis types.

Episcleritis is an acute, localized, self-limited inflammation of the episclera, presenting with a mild pink to red eye. Pain is typically absent, although mild discomfort may be experienced. Slit-lamp examination reveals injection of superficial blood vessels confined to the episcleral tissue (Figure 17-2). The inflammation vanishes with 10% phenylephrine drops. Recurrences are common but decrease in frequency after 4 years. Up to 32% of patients have an underlying systemic disorder (Table 17-1).

What Are the Likely Etiologies of Scleritis?

An underlying systemic disorder is present in approximately 60% of patients with scleritis (see Table 17-1). Connective tissue or vasculitic diseases are present in nearly 48% of patients; 10% have an infectious etiology; and 2% have atopy, rosacea, or gout.[1,2] Rheumatoid arthritis (RA) and Wegener's granulomatosis (WG) are the most common systemic associations, followed by relapsing polychondritis, systemic lupus erythematosus (SLE), and arthritis with inflammatory bowel disease.[1] The incidence of scleritis in patients with RA is almost 7%,[1] and up to 4% of patients have WG, a potentially fatal, multisystem disorder. Necrotizing scleritis, which is associated with an increased risk of mortality, is a common subtype observed in both diseases.[3]

Presence of scleritis is a reasonably accurate guide to systemic activity in a patient with SLE. Sclerotic attacks become aggressive and recurrent as the disease deteriorates and resolve with adequate control of SLE.

Ankylosing spondylitis (AS) has a strong association with HLA-B27 and tendency for ocular inflammation. AS scleritis generally takes the form of diffuse scleritis, which, despite recurrences, rarely progresses to necrotizing scleritis.[2]

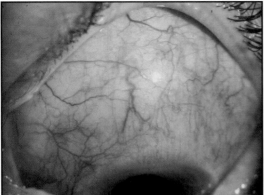

Figure 17-2. Episcleritis. Note the pinkish hue with injection and dilation of the superficial episcleral blood vessels.

Table 17-1

Associated Conditions in Episcleritis and Scleritis

Noninfectious	*Infectious*
Connective tissue diseases • Rheumatoid arthritis • Systemic lupus erythematosus • Seronegative spondyloarthropathies • Ankylosing spondylitis • Reiter's syndrome • Psoriatic arthritis • Arthritis and inflammatory bowel disease • Relapsing polychondritis	**Bacteria** • Gram positive and gram negative • Mycobacteria • Spirochetes • Chlamydia • Actinomyces • Nocardia
Vasculitides • Wegener's granulomatosis • Polyarteritis nodosa • Churg-Strauss syndrome • Behcet's disease • Giant cell arteritis • Cogan's syndrome	**Viruses** • Herpes zoster • Herpes simplex • Mumps
	Fungi • Filamentous fungi • Dimorphic fungi
	Parasites • Acanthamoeba
Miscellaneous • Atopy • Rosacea • Gout • Foreign body granuloma • Trauma—chemical and/or physical injury • Postsurgical • Drugs	**Toxoplasmosis** • Toxocariasis

Psoriatic arthritis (PA) is a triad of psoriasis, inflammatory arthritis, and a negative test for rheumatoid factor. Nail pitting is nearly pathognomonic for the disease. Incidence of scleritis in patients with PA is 1.8%, occurring after years of active arthritis. Although diffuse scleritis is often seen, it may take almost any form.[1,2]

Gastrointestinal and articular manifestations are the hallmarks of inflammatory bowel disease (IBD). Scleritis occurs in 10% of patients with IBD, occurs some years after the onset of intestinal symptoms, and is more common in patients with extraintestinal manifestations.

Although immune-mediated diseases are the main disorders associated with scleritis, less common etiologies such as infections should also be considered. Infectious agents cause scleritis through direct invasion or an immune response and should be suspected in cases of indolent progressive scleral necrosis, especially if the past history reveals trauma, chronic topical steroid use, surgical procedures, or systemic disease.

Infections with organisms such as pseudomonas, herpes, or tuberculosis cause severe scleritis that is difficult to treat. Although rare, herpes simplex virus infections and malignancies occasionally masquerade as scleritis and, thus, are essential to rule out in patients presenting with scleritis of unknown etiology unresponsive to conventional therapy.

How Should This Patient Be Worked Up?

Scleritis may be the initial or only presenting clinical manifestation of several potentially fatal disorders. The correct and rapid diagnosis and appropriate therapy are essential to halt the relentless progression of both ocular and systemic processes, preventing globe destruction and possibly saving the patient's life. A detailed past history, review of systems (ROS), and physical examination along with appropriate diagnostic tests (Table 17-2) are imperative to confirm or reject any suspected systemic disorder.

In RA, checking for rheumatoid factor (RF) testing including IgG and IgA RF (see Table 17-2) in addition to IgM RF is appropriate in any patient with scleritis who has arthralgias. In WG, detection of antineutrophil cytoplasmic antibodies (ANCA) is the initial and most crucial serologic test along with urine analysis with microscopy and chest and sinus imaging (computed tomography).[3] Patients with scleritis who are ANCA-positive have aggressive disease and must be treated accordingly. Ocular tissue biopsy may be indicated in some cases of scleritis associated with an underlying systemic condition, in order to establish diagnosis, or in cases of recurrent or refractory scleritis.

How Should This Patient Be Treated?

Episcleritis, a self-limiting disease, requires no treatment. Some patients may benefit from the use of artificial tears and oral nonsteroidal anti-inflammatory drugs (NSAIDs). Topical NSAIDs may help in some instances, and while topical steroids may seem like magic, it is an unwise approach because this strategy can prolong the total duration of the patient's problem.

Table 17-2

Systemic Disorders Associated With Scleritis and Their Relevant Diagnostic Tests

	RF	ANCA	ANA	CIC	C	Cryo	X-ray	HLA	Ig	U/A	HBsAg	WBC	BUN & CrCl	ESR/CRP	Urate	Ser
Ankylosing Spondylitis	-	-	-	+	-	-	sacro-iliac	+	-	-	-	-	-	-	-	-
Atopy	-	-	-	-	-	-	chest	-	E	-	-	Eo	-	-	-	-
Behcet's	-	-	-	+	+	-	-	+	-	-	-	-	-	-	-	-
Churg-Strauss	-	-	-	+	-	-	chest	-	E	-	-	Eo	-	-	-	-
Cogan's syndrome	-	-	-	+	+	-		-	-	-	-	-		-	-	-
Giant cell arteritis	-	-	-	+	-	-	-	-	G	-	-	-	-	+	-	-
Gout	-	-	-	-	-	-	limb	-	-	-	-	-	-	-	+	-
IBD arthritis	-	-	-	-	-	-	limb, sacro-iliac & abdominal	-	-	-	-	-				
Infectious	-	-	-	-	-	-	-	-	-	-	-	-	-	-	-	+
PAN	-	-	-	+	+	+	-	-	-	+	+	-	-	-	-	-
Psoriatic arthritis	-	-	-	-	-	-	limb & sacro-iliac	-	-	-	-	-	-	-	-	-

(continued)

Table 17-2 (continued)

Systemic Disorders Associated With Scleritis and Their Relevant Diagnostic Tests

	RF	ANCA	ANA	CIC	C	Cryo	X-ray	HLA	Ig	U/A	HBsAg	WBC	BUN & CrCl	ESR/ CRP	Urate	Ser
RA	+	-	Anti-DNA his-tone	+	+	+	limb joints	+	-	-	-	-	-	-	-	-
Reiter's	-	-	-	+	-	-	sacro-iliac	+	-	+	-	-	-	-	-	-
Relapsing polychon-dritis	-	-	-	+	+	-	-	-	-	-	-	-	-	-	-	-
SLE	-	-	Anti-ds DNA;													
Anti-Sm Ag	+	+	+	-	-	·G	+	-	-	-	-	-	-	-	-	
Wegener's	+	+	-	+	-	-	chest & sinus	-	A; E	+	-	-	+	-	-	-

"+": Test significantly warranted for investigation   "-": Test may or may not be warranted for diagnosis

RF, rheumatoid factor; ANCA, antineutrophil cytoplasmic antibodies; ANA, antinuclear antibodies; CIC, circulating immune complex; C, complement (C3 and C4); Cryo, cryoglobulin; HLA, human leukocyte antigen (HLA typing); Ig, immunoglobulin; U/A, urinanalysis; HBsAg, hepatitis B surface antigen; WBC, white blood cell count; BUN, blood urea nitrogen; CrCl, creatinine clearance; ESR, erythrocyte segmentation rate; IBD, inflammatory bowel disease; RA, rheumatoid arthritis; SLE, systemic lupus erythematosus; PAN, polyarteritis nodosa; anti-ds DNA, anti-double stranded DNA; anti-Sm Ag, anti-smith antigen; Eo, eosinophils.

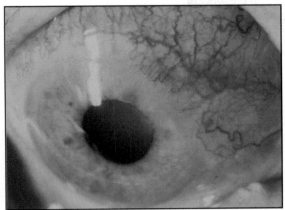

Figure 17-3. Diffuse scleritis. Note the redness with violaceous hue and dilation and injection of the deep episcleral blood vessels.

Treatment of scleritis is streamlined to target any underlying systemic disorder, achieve the desired response, and minimize the side effects of therapy. Patients generally do not respond well to topical medications and require systemic therapy with NSAIDs, steroids, or other immunosuppressive drugs. Oral NSAIDs are the first line of treatment for non-necrotizing anterior scleritis. Up to one-third of patients with diffuse (Figure 17-3) and two-thirds of patients with nodular scleritis respond well to oral NSAIDs within 3 weeks.

Patients with necrotizing (Figure 17-4) and non-necrotizing scleritis with associated systemic disorder are not likely to respond to oral NSAIDs alone. They require steroids at a dose of 1 mg/kg/day, tapered slowly upon clinical remission at the rate of 10 mg/week until 5 mg/day is reached. This is essential to prevent bone loss and other inevitable complications associated with long-term steroid use.

Immunosuppressants are used in case of failure to respond to high-dose steroids or if unacceptably high doses of steroids are needed to maintain remission. This allows a lower dose of steroids to achieve quiescence, hence, decreasing the risk of side effects. Up to 25% of patients require treatment with steroid-sparing drugs for long-term control of disease, especially patients with necrotizing scleritis or underlying systemic disorder.

One of the best initial choices of immunosuppressants is methotrexate at a dose of 15 to 30 mg/week, which is efficacious, has a more favorable side effect profile and has lower oncogenic potential as compared to alkylating agents. Azathioprine 2 mg/kg/day or mycophenolate mofetil 1 g twice daily is also effective. Alkylating agents, such as cyclophosphamide 2 mg/kg/day, along with steroids, are used as a last line effort or as a first line therapy in patients with WG or PAN.

Alternately, intravenous high-dose methylprednisolone 1 g/day 3 times within the first week, with dose reduction weekly thereafter, can be used with or without immunosuppressive agents. The use of periocular injection of steroids for non-necrotizing scleritis has been limited by side effects, including increased intraocular pressure, cataract formation, exacerbation of scleral melting, and globe perforation.[4]

Current research is focused on the use of biologics; these are monoclonal antibodies (MAB) such as infliximab (tumor necrosis factor alpha inhibitor), daclizumab (IgG monoclonal antibody which binds to CD25 of IL-2 receptor), and rituximab (anti-CD20 B-cell monoclonal antibody) used in the treatment of scleritis.

Figure 17-4. Necrotizing scleritis. Note not only the loss of sclera and pronounced avascularity of the necrotized area, but also the surrounding inflammatory signs.

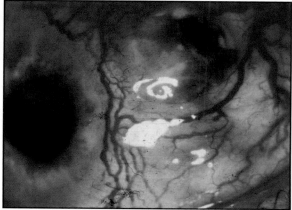

References

1. Foster CS, Sainz de la Maza M. *The sclera*. New York, NY: Springer-Verlag; 1994.
2. Watson PG, Hayreh SS. Scleritis and episcleritis. *Br J Ophthalmol*. 1976;60:163-191.
3. Joshi L, Hamour S, Salama AD, et al. Renal and ocular targets for therapy in Wegener's granulomatosis. *Inflamm Allergy Drug Targets*. 2009;8(1):70-79.
4. Jabs D, Mudun A, Dunn J, et al. Episcleritis and scleritis: clinical features and treatment results. *Am J Ophthalmol*. 2000;130:469-476.

AN 18-YEAR-OLD MALE COMPLAINING OF SEVERE ITCHY EYES AND REDNESS HAS DIFFUSE EYELID ERYTHEMA WITH DRY SCALY SKIN, MEIBOMIAN GLAND DYSFUNCTION, 2+ CONJUNCTIVAL BULBAR AND PALPEBRAL INJECTION, AND 3+ PAPILLAE. DOES HE NEED STEROID DROPS?

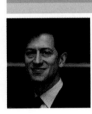

Michael B. Raizman, MD

Vernal conjunctivitis is a condition of children and teenagers that rarely continues into adulthood. While it can be associated with generalized atopy, some patients have no other allergic manifestations. Vernal can have many presentations, but a classic version involves severe itching of both eyes in the springtime, associated with giant papillae of the upper tarsal or limbal conjunctiva. The disease can have periods of remission or can be chronic and may be seasonal. With chronic inflammation, corneal ulceration and vascularization can develop. The 18-year-old patient described in this case has significant eyelid skin inflammation without typical ocular surface changes of vernal conjunctivitis. This patient would fall into the category of atopic conjunctivitis and blepharitis rather than vernal conjunctivitis (Figure 18-1). The management strategies are similar for atopic and vernal conjunctivitis, but atopic disease can continue into adulthood and progress over time. Therefore, the prognosis can be worse with atopic disease.

Figure 18-1. Severe atopic blepharitis associated with diffuse eczema and chronic allergic conjunctivitis.

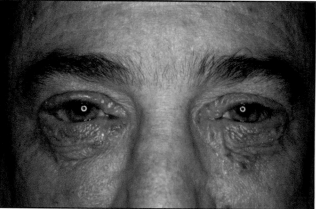

Management

   The fundamental management of any patient with atopic disease is to recognize possible environmental contributors and educate the patient on avoidance. Allergists can be helpful in the management of these patients, even if the disease is only in and around the eyes. If patients have ongoing exposure to environmental allergens, it may be impossible to control the ocular signs and symptoms. Another fundamental principle of management is educating the patient on the detrimental consequences of eye rubbing. Touching the eyes and face can bring allergens and environmental irritants in contact with the skin, nose, and conjunctiva. In addition, the mechanical force of eye rubbing can induce degranulation of mast cells. This has been demonstrated to worsen allergic symptoms.[1] Many cases of eczema of the skin develop only with mechanical irritation. Elimination of rubbing and scratching can eliminate the eczema in these cases. Patients with allergic conjunctivitis of any cause will have ocular itching. If patients rub their eyes, they can develop lid skin changes. The corollary of this is patients with eczema of the lid skin who develop conjunctival swelling and itching after rubbing the eyes, because the lid skin itches. If patients continue to touch and rub their eyes, it may be impossible to control their signs and symptoms with medical therapy.

   After patients have been educated about avoidance of allergens and the importance of keeping the hands away from the face, medication can be prescribed to help with the signs and symptoms. We are fortunate to have many highly effective and safe topical agents for treating conjunctivitis. Topical mast cell stabilizers, antihistamines, and combination agents are usually effective. Topical corticosteroids can be used for more severe cases. Loteprednol may be the safest steroid for chronic use because it is less likely to induce cataract formation and glaucoma, but all steroids need to be used with caution and with careful observation. Topical corticosteroids are usually mandatory when the cornea becomes involved with any allergic condition. Severe ocular allergy can be blinding, and aggressive therapy is warranted for corneal involvement.[2]

   Treatment of eczema of the eyelid skin can be challenging. Patients should be instructed to avoid application of cosmetics, lotions, creams, and soaps to the eyelid skin. Eyelid scrubs should be avoided in any patient with eczema. Consultation with an allergist can help identify allergens. Eyelid skin inflammation can be triggered by hand care products and jewelry. Hand lotions, nail polish, nail polish remover, and metal rings and bracelets have been demonstrated to cause eczema on the lid skin. This may occur because the skin on the eyelids is especially thin and may be especially susceptible to inflammation.

Application of topical corticosteroids to the lid skin can be helpful. In general, it is best to avoid fluorinated corticosteroids on the lid skin because of their propensity to thin the skin. I advise against use of products such as fluorometholone or tobramycin/ dexamethasone ointment on the lid skin. Hydrocortisone 0.5% or 1% cream is available over the counter and can be used safely for 1 or 2 weeks, once or twice a day. Even with these less potent topical corticosteroids, patients must be advised of the risks of chronic application. Dermatologists often prescribe desonide lotion for use on the face, and this can be used safely on the eyelid skin. For chronic therapy, I prescribe pimecrolimus (Elidel) or tacrolimus (Protopic) once or twice a day.[3] This is safe to use on the lid skin even though the package insert advises against it. Some patients will experience burning and stinging if the product gets into the eye. In this case, they should rinse the eye with artificial tears. They should be careful not to apply the medication too close to the lid margin. There have been reports of possible induction of tumors with chronic use of topical cyclosporine derivatives. I mention this to my patients when I prescribe pimecrolimus. The development of tumors is extremely rare and is probably associated with use of these medications over a large part of the body in patients with generalized eczema rather than application to the eyelid skin.

References

1. Raizman MB, Rothman JS, Maroun F, Rand WM. Effect of eye rubbing on signs and symptoms of allergic conjunctivitis in cat-sensitive individuals. *Curr Allergy Asthma Rep.* 2002;2(4):319-320.
2. Foster CS, Calonge M. Atopic keratoconjunctivitis. *Ophthalmology.* 1990;97(8):992-1000.
3. Williams HC, Grindlay DJ. What's new in atopic eczema? An analysis of the clinical significance of systematic reviews on atopic eczema published in 2006 and 2007. *Clin Exp Dermatol.* 2008;33(6):685-688.

A 72-Year-Old Female Has Conjunctival Injection in Both Eyes and Symblepharon and Trichiasis in the Right Eye. The Right Cornea Has Moderate Punctate Staining. Should I Just Pull Out the Lashes or Do a Wedge Resection of the Lower Lid to Tighten It Up?

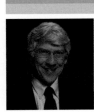

David D. Verdier, MD

The answer is neither. The trichiasis needs proper treatment, but it is not this patient's major concern. The red flag in her exam, in flashing neon lights, is the finding of symblepharon. The most common and feared diagnosis associated with symblepharon is mucous membrane pemphigoid (MMP), also known as ocular cicatricial pemphigoid. Untreated, MMP often leads to blindness and can even lead to death from pharyngeal or esophageal stricture. Even with proper treatment, up to 50% of patients with MMP have progressive conjunctival cicatrization and vision loss.

Etiology, Course, and Treatment of Mucous Membrane Pemphigoid

MMP is an immune-related progressive systemic disease that affects the mucous membranes of the eye, nose, mouth, respiratory and gastrointestinal tracts, and skin. It is characterized by linear deposition of immunoglobulins and/or complement in the basement membrane, causing subepithelial blistering and cicatrization. Ocular involvement is present in up to 80% of MMP patients.[1] Approximately 50% of MMP patients with ocular involvement have non-ocular systemic findings, such as mouth and nasopharyngeal vesicobullous lesions, esophageal strictures, cutaneous blisters, and erythematous plaques.[2]

Ocular MMP is usually bilateral. It most often occurs between age 30 and 90 with peak involvement in the seventh decade. There is a slight female preponderance.

Signs of ocular MMP include chronic, often episodic conjunctivitis, which is a sign of active disease. Subepithelial fibrosis causes conjunctival foreshortening, which can progress to symblepharon and often entropion and trichiasis. Meibomian gland and lacrimal ductule obstruction cause dry eye problems, often contributing to corneal ulceration, scarring, and neovascularization. In end-stage disease, the cornea can become opacified and keratinized, and the lids fused.

Patients with active autoimmune-driven conjunctival inflammation require systemic immunosuppression to limit disease progression. Topical steroids are of little value. Because of the considerable morbidity, mortality, and long-term expense of systemic immunosuppression, strong consideration should be given for the patient to have mucous membrane or skin biopsy with immunohistochemistry studies demonstrating IgG, IgA, or complement components along the basement membrane zone. However, negative or inconclusive biopsy results do not exclude the diagnosis of MMP in the presence of characteristic clinical features.

Differential Diagnosis for Cicatrizing Conjunctivitis

MMP is often a diagnosis of exclusion. Our patient requires a thorough history and physical exam, including review of systems. The differential diagnosis of cicatrizing conjunctivitis includes past lid surgery or trauma, radiation, chemical or thermal burns, Stevens-Johnson syndrome, Sjögren's syndrome, trachoma, atopic keratoconjunctivitis, post-infectious conjunctivitis, rosacea, graft-versus-host disease, lichen planus, conjunctival squamous or sebaceous cell carcinoma, and paraneoplastic pseudopemphigoid. An association between chronic use of glaucoma medications and cicatrizing conjunctivitis has also been referred to as pseudopemphigoid.

The first order of business in our patient is to establish her diagnosis. A careful history and physical exam should rule in or out most non-MMP causes of cicatrizing conjunctivitis. Does the patient have a positive history of esophageal stricture or problems swallowing? Does she have any skin or oral mucosa findings? What are the frequency, duration, and clinical findings of her conjunctivitis? Look for subtle evidence of cicatrization in either eye assisted by successively pulling each lid away from the field of gaze (Figure 19-1). Some corneal consultants believe any patient with a history suggestive of MMP should be biopsied. However, biopsy is not without risk, as disrupting the conjunctiva in a patient with cicatrizing conjunctivitis may cause flare-up of the disease. Oral mucosa lesions may offer a less risky biopsy site. I may hold off on biopsy especially if the disease appears quiet, in which case I may also hold off on treatment. Furthermore, if the disease presentation is strongly consistent with the diagnosis of MMP, I might skip the biopsy as I will likely initiate treatment even if the biopsy is negative, given the 20% chance of a false negative result.

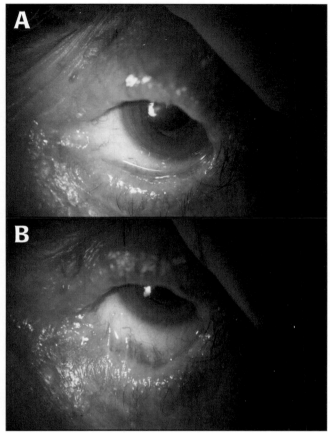

Figure 19-1. Difficult-to-appreciate cicatrization in primary gaze (A). Cicatrization easily demonstrated with retracting lower lid inferiorly with same eye in upgaze (B).

Management

Our 72-year-old patient has active bilateral conjunctival involvement that has progressed to the point of symblepharon formation. In the absence of likely explanation for a non-MMP etiology, she needs a biopsy and very likely prompt systemic immunosuppressive therapy. A team approach is optimal, including an ophthalmologist to follow ocular disease activity and progression and a specialist (usually an oncologist, rheumatologist, or dermatologist) with experience in systemic immunosuppressive therapy. Treatment should be tailored to each patient with a step-wise approach (Table 19-1).[2,3] At each visit, I like to grade and record conjunctival injection in each quadrant to document the degree of active ocular disease. Disease progression can be measured by staging based on the extent of conjunctival foreshortening and symblepharon (Table 19-2).[4]

The treatment plan must also include supportive care for the ocular surface, including aggressive dry eye and blepharitis treatment and correction of lid anomalies including trichiasis. Trichiasis in patients with MMP is often associated with entropion formation. Adhering to the team approach for this very serious disease, I would refer our patient to an oculoplastic consultant. He or she might advocate a lid-splitting technique with or without mucous membrane grafting to treat both entropion and misdirected lashes, with care to minimize conjunctival disruption.[5] Wedge resection is less desirable for our

---

Table 19-1
MMP Treatment Options

Mild to moderate disease: Dapsone; alternatives: sulfapyridine, methotrexate
Moderate disease: Mycophenalate mofetil or azathioprine
Severe disease: Cyclophosphamide plus short-course oral steroids
Refractory disease: Consider IV immunoglobulin

All patients:
- Consider combination therapy
- Co-manage with oncologist, rheumatologist, or dermatologist

---

Table 19-2
Staging of MMP

Stage I.   Subepithelial fibrosis and inflammation of conjunctiva
Stage II.   Shrinkage of conjunctiva with foreshortening of fornices
Stage III. Symblepharon formation
Stage IV.   Ankyloblepharon formation

---

patient as it adds to conjunctival shortening and may involve more direct conjunctival contact. Manual epilation offers no long-term solution. Trichiasis should include a more permanent approach such as electrocautery or radiofrequency ablation.

Corneal transplantation should be avoided in most MMP patients because of the very high risk of failure from both ocular surface compromise and rejection. I would consider corneal transplantation or keratoprosthesis as a last resort, and only if vision loss is bilateral and severe.

Should our patient develop significant cataract, she will likely do well with cataract surgery as long as the eye is quiet and a clear corneal incision approach is used. Control of MMP by immunosuppressive therapy should be optimized prior to cataract surgery, and it can be augmented by a perioperative course of oral or intravenous steroids (eg, a 10-day course of oral prednisone 60 mg daily starting 3 days prior to surgery).

References

1. Thorne JE, Anhalt GJ, Jabs DA. Mucous membrane pemphigoid and pseudopemphigoid. *Ophthalmology.* 2004;111:45-52.
2. Saw VP, Dart JK, Rauz S, et al. Immunosuppressive therapy for ocular mucous membrane pemphigoid. *Ophthalmology.* 2008;115:253-261.
3. Thorne JE, Woreta FA, Jabs DA, et al. Treatment of ocular mucous membrane pemphigoid with immunosuppressive drug therapy. *Ophthalmology.* 2008;115:2146-2152.
4. Foster CS. Cicatricial pemphigoid. *Trans Am Ophthalmol Soc.* 1986;84:527-663.
5. Koreen IV, Taich A, Elner VM. Anterior lamellar recession with buccal mucous membrane grafting for cicatricial entropion. *Ophthal Plast Reconstr Surg.* 2009;25:180-184.

A 67-YEAR-OLD FEMALE COMPLAINS OF CONSTANT EYE IRRITATION. THE EXAM SHOWS CONJUNCTIVOCHALASIS OF THE LOWER BULBAR CONJUNCTIVA. SHOULD I EXCISE THE REDUNDANT CONJUNCTIVA?

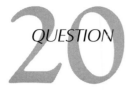

James P. Dunn, MD
(co-authored with Aarup A. Kubal, MD)

Conjunctivochalasis is characterized by lax, redundant bulbar conjunctiva (Figure 20-1), usually located inferiorly and overhanging the lower lid margin. The condition is almost always bilateral but may be asymmetric. Clinically diagnosed on the basis of slit-lamp examination, it is usually found in the temporal conjunctiva and lacks edema, thus distinguishing it from the chemosis characteristic of allergic conjunctivitis. Much like dermatochalasis, or redundancy of eyelid skin, conjunctivochalasis is found in association with aging and has been regarded as a normal change in aging individuals.

Mild cases may be asymptomatic, but patients often complain of foreign body sensation, burning, tearing, and blurry vision. These are symptoms typical of dry eye, and it has been suggested that the redundant conjunctiva may worsen aqueous tear deficiency by interfering with the normal tear meniscus and further destabilizing the tear film. Epiphora can result from interference with the tear film or obstruction of the inferior punctum by redundant folds of conjunctiva, resulting in delayed tear clearance. In more severe cases, rubbing of the conjunctival folds against themselves and the lid margins may cause subconjunctival hemorrhage. Excessive conjunctivochalasis may even result in nocturnal lagophthalmos by mechanically obstructing eyelid closure. This severe presentation may be accompanied by Dellen formation or exposure keratopathy.[1]

Figure 20-1. Note the redundant superior conjunctiva easily induced with gentle eyelid closure. The patient was bothered by chronic irritation and foreign body sensation.

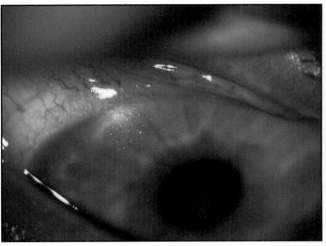

What Causes Conjunctivochalasis?

The cause of conjunctivochalasis is unknown. The increased prevalence of conjunctivochalasis with age suggests that age-related changes in the stiffness of the conjunctiva and its attachment to the underlying Tenon's and sclera may be involved. Although conjunctival specimens from histopathologic studies of conjunctivochalasis are usually normal, the presence of elastosis has been reported. Furthermore, fibroblasts cultured from conjunctivochalasis specimens have been shown to have increased expression of matrix metalloproteinases, particularly MMP-1 and MMP-3. This finding may be associated with increased collagenolytic activity and degradation of the conjunctival extracellular matrix.[2] Whether sun exposure and UV radiation trigger these degenerative changes has not been established.

Another potential trigger for the development of conjunctivochalasis is mechanical trauma. Over time, repeated microtrauma, either from eye rubbing or blinking, may weaken the conjunctival stroma or disrupt the conjunctival attachment to Tenon's capsule. This theory is further supported by a recent study that links contact lens wear, particularly hard contact lens wear, with the presence and severity of conjunctivochalasis.[3] Repeated friction from the contact lens against the conjunctiva likely induces microtrauma that weakens the conjunctival stroma and contributes to conjunctival laxity. Hypoxia and chronic inflammation may also contribute.

The role of inflammation, however, is controversial. Earlier reports of conjunctivochalasis suggested that inflammation played a minimal role, if any, in the pathogenesis of conjunctivochalasis while more recent reports have linked the 2. Clinicopathologic studies are inconsistent, with some demonstrating no difference between conjunctivochalasis specimens and normal controls and others showing a subset of patients with signs of inflammation. In a recent histopathologic study, 4 of 29 (14%) conjunctivochalasis specimens demonstrated a sub-epithelial chronic inflammatory infiltrate consisting of plasma cells and lymphocytes.[2] Furthermore, inflammatory cytokines, including interleukin 1b (IL-1b) and tumor necrosis factor α (TNFα), have been demonstrated in higher concentrations in tear samples from patients with chalatic conjunctiva versus normal controls.[4] That only a small subset of patients demonstrates inflammatory changes suggests that the underlying etiology of conjunctivochalasis is multifactorial.

How Is Conjunctivochalasis Diagnosed?

Because conjunctivochalasis is common, especially in the elderly, and because associated conditions such as keratoconjunctivitis sicca present with similar symptoms, conjunctivochalasis is an often overlooked ocular surface disorder. In the evaluation of patients with irritation and tearing, a careful slit-lamp exam must be performed, looking for lid laxity and/or malposition, punctal stenosis or ectropion, and trichiasis or distichiasis. The nature of the tear meniscus and the presence of fluorescein and/or rose bengal staining should also be documented. Supplemental investigations, including Schirmer's testing to evaluate for tear deficiency and lacrimal irrigation to rule out nasolacrimal duct obstruction, may be of benefit.

What Are the Medical and Surgical Treatment Options?

Treatment of conjunctivochalasis should be guided by patients' symptoms. Asymptomatic conjunctivochalasis needs no treatment. Mildly symptomatic cases with foreign body sensation or burning as the main complaints may benefit from a trial of artificial tears and lubricating ointments. This intervention, however, is unlikely to help—and may even worsen symptoms—in patients suffering from epiphora. Topical corticosteroids or antihistamines/mast cell stabilizers are of little benefit.

In severe cases, surgical correction to remove redundant conjunctiva should be considered. The surgical approach usually involves isolating the conjunctiva to be excised with a forceps 3- to 5-mm posterior to the inferior limbus. An elliptical or crescent-shaped area, measuring approximately 3- to 5-mm wide and 10- to 12-mm long, is then marked. Anesthesia is achieved with a subconjunctival injection of lidocaine with epinephrine, the redundant conjunctiva is resected, and closure is achieved with absorbable sutures. Care should be taken to avoid excessive conjunctival resection as this may lead to scarring, posterior lamellar shortening, and cicatricial entropion. An alternative to this procedure that is especially useful in cases of conjunctivochalasis overhanging the central part of the lower eyelid involves creating a 90-degree peritomy centered at the 6 o'clock meridian. Radial relaxing incisions are then made at the medial and temporal edges of the peritomy, and the conjunctiva is undermined and advanced superiorly over the cornea. Redundant conjunctiva is then trimmed at the limbus, and conjunctival closure is obtained with absorbable sutures. Favorable results have been obtained using amniotic membrane transplants, either sutured in place or affixed with fibrin glue over the area of conjunctival resection. This approach may increase adherence of the conjunctiva to underlying structures and reduce conjunctival laxity.[1]

References

1. Meller D, Tseng SCG. Conjunctivochalasis: literature review and possible pathophysiology. *Surv Ophthalmol.* 1998;43:225-232.
2. Francis C, Chan DG, Kim P, et al. Case-controlled clinical and histopathological study of conjunctivochalasis. *Br J Ophthalmol.* 2005;89:302-305.
3. Mimura T, Usui T, Yamamoto H, et al. Conjunctivochalasis and contact lenses. *Am J Ophthalmol.* 2009;148(1):20-25.
4. Wang Y, Dogru M, Matsumoto Y, et al. The impact of nasal conjunctivochalasis on tear functions and ocular surface findings. *Am J Ophthalmol.* 2007;144:930-937.

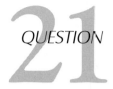

A Patient Complaining of Eye Irritation Has Moderate Meibomian Gland Dysfunction and Trace Conjunctival Injection. Could This Be Rosacea?

Richard E. Braunstein, MD
(co-authored with Prathima R. Thumma, MD)

Rosacea is a chronic, inflammatory skin condition that affects the facial area, including the nose, forehead, cheeks, and chin. It is seen in middle-aged adults of all races but is more frequently diagnosed in fair-skinned individuals. Although it is more prevalent in women, rosacea can be more severe in men. It is characterized by facial flushing, erythema, telangiectasias, pustules, papules, and rhinophyma (Figure 21-1). Rosacea frequently involves the eye and affects mostly the eyelids and ocular surface. Primary features of ocular rosacea are blepharitis and conjunctivitis. Hordeola, chalazia, superficial punctate keratopathy, recurrent corneal erosions, corneal vascularization, corneal infiltrates, corneal perforation, iritis, episcleritis, and scleritis related to rosacea have also been reported.[1,2]

Because rosacea affects sebaceous glands, ocular rosacea is primarily a dysfunction of meibomian glands (Figure 21-2). Chronic inflammation of the lid margin results in changes in the anatomy of the glands and the composition of their secretions. This results in plugged, pouting meibomian glands with thick lipid secretions and foamy tears. Symptoms include burning, itching, irritation, foreign body sensation, and blurry vision. Longstanding disease may be associated with corneal epithelial keratopathy, neovascularization, pannus, marginal infiltrates, and phlyctenules.[1]

Figure 21-1. Rhinophyma with facial telangiectasias.

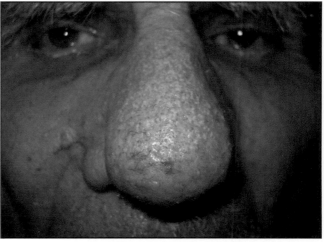

Figure 21-2. Rosacea blepharitis with meibomian gland congestion and lid margin inflammation.

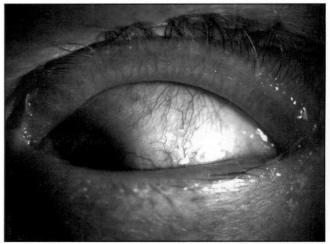

Management

Ocular rosacea is a bilateral, chronic, recurrent disease with a waxing and waning course. Therefore, the goal of treatment is tailored to the patient's symptoms. In this case, the symptoms are relatively mild; therefore, treatment should first start with lid hygiene and artificial tears. The patient should apply a washcloth soaked in warm water on closed eyelids for about 5 minutes. Warm compresses help to soften and liquefy the secretions from the meibomian glands. This should be followed by digital massage of the lid margins to express these secretions and gentle cleansing of the eye with a non-irritating solution, such as commercial eyelid scrubs or a 50/50 mixture of water and baby shampoo, to remove any debris. Preservative-free artificial tears should be used frequently during the day and a lubricating ointment at night, if needed.

If the condition persists despite conservative measures, oral antibiotics should be considered. Oral tetracyclines (eg, tetracycline, doxycycline, minocycline) are quite effective in the treatment of rosacea. They are not used for their antibiotic properties but rather for their action on the meibomian glands. Tetracyclines alter the composition of the meibomian secretions by decreasing lipase production by both S. epidermidis and S. aureus. This results in increased solubility of these secretions and greater tear film stability.[3] Oral tetracyclines are contraindicated in pregnant or nursing women.

Doxycycline 100 mg twice a day can be used for 3 weeks and then tapered to a dose of 100 mg once a day for 2 to 3 months, depending on the severity of the condition and the response to the medication. Because the antibiotic property is not the primary consideration, low-dose doxycycline 20 mg should strongly be considered where chronic therapy is warranted. Tetracycline may be started at 250 mg 4 times a day, and then tapered after 3 weeks. It is very important to warn patients of increased photosensitivity while using these medications. The use of sunscreen is crucial, especially during the summer months. Patients with gastrointestinal side effects of tetracycline can often tolerate enteric-coated doxycycline. It generally takes several weeks to see some therapeutic effect. Erythromycin and clarithromycin can be used as alternatives in patients with a history of hypersensitivity to tetracyclines or intolerable side effects.

The use of topical corticosteroids should be reserved for short-term management of inflammation including marginal keratitis, phlyctenules, or severe conjunctival injection. The lowest dose of corticosteroids that will control the symptoms with a tapering course should be used. Corneal involvement may suggest worsening eye disease. In the presence of superficial punctate keratitis (SPK), treatment should start with lid hygiene, frequent (q1h) administration of preservative-free artificial tears, and lubricating ointment at bedtime with a low-threshold for use of low-dose tetracycline because of their anti-collagenase properties.

Staphylococcal marginal keratitis is also seen in conjunction with chronic blepharitis. It is a hypersensitivity reaction to staphylococcal antigens and is characterized by focal, sterile, sub-epithelial infiltrates. These non-staining lesions are located at the peripheral cornea and are separated from the limbus by a peripheral clear zone. Mild topical corticosteroids alone or in combination with an antibiotic are very effective in the treatment of this condition.

Unlike staphylococcal marginal keratitis described above, rosacea-related keratitis has been described as grayish-white sub-epithelial infiltrates with vascular infiltration (Figure 21-3). These lesions typically extend from the limbus inferiorly toward the central cornea. Ulceration, thinning, and corneal perforation may occur if not treated appropriately.[1] Ocular involvement usually follows dermatologic findings, but occasionally, the patient may first present with eye findings.[2,4] There does not appear to be any consensus on the natural history of rosacea keratitis and facial rosacea. Some authors note that skin and eye findings are independent of each other while others describe a tendency for both conditions to flare up at the same time.[2] It is important to note that oral isotretinoin, which is quite effective in reducing the inflammation of facial rosacea, can exacerbate blepharoconjunctivitis and even cause severe keratitis.[1,2]

Figure 21-3. Rosacea keratitis with superficial vascularization and corneal scarring.

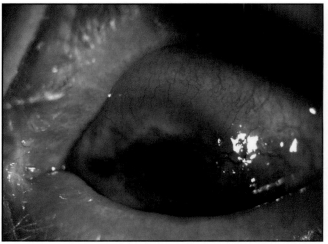

References

1. American Academy of Ophthalmology, Ophthalmic News and Education Network. *Blepharitis: Preferred Practice Pattern Guideline.* 2008. Available at: http://one.aao.org/CE/PracticeGuidelines/PPP.aspx. Accessed May 4, 2009.
2. Browning DJ, Proia AD. Ocular rosacea. *Surv Ophthalmol.* 1986;31(3):145-158.
3. Jackson WB. Blepharitis: current strategies for diagnosis and management. *Can J Ophthalmol.* 2008;43(2):170-179.
4. Krachmer JH, Mannis MJ, Holland EJ. *Cornea: Fundamentals, Diagnosis and Management (Vol 1).* 2nd ed. Philadelphia, PA: Mosby; 2005.

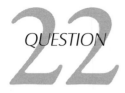

QUESTION 22

A 49-YEAR-OLD MALE COMES TO THE OFFICE WITH A RED SWOLLEN UPPER EYELID. THE SYMPTOMS STARTED YESTERDAY. SHOULD I START TREATING HIM FOR CHALAZION?

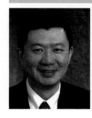

John D. Ng, MD, MS, FACS

A hordeolum is an acutely inflamed, blocked sebaceous gland of the eyelid due either to infection or local inflammation from leakage of sebaceous material out of the gland structure and into the surrounding tissue. Hordeola may be anterior involving the glands of Zeiss or, more commonly, posterior involving the meibomian glands in the tarsus. A chalazion is a posterior hordeolum that can either be acute (ie, inflamed) or chronic (ie, quiet and non-inflamed). Acute chalazia or hordeola are usually painful and tender to palpation and may suppurate and spontaneously drain. Chronic chalazia are usually encapsulated and non-tender and cause symptoms due to mass effect. Because they are encapsulated, chronic chalazia usually do not spontaneously drain, but take many months to resorb.

Clinical Presentation and Initial Treatment

If a patient presents with acute onset of an inflamed, red eyelid, infection such as a preseptal cellulitis must be ruled out. If there is no nidus of inflammation or swollen meibomian gland, but there is diffuse inflammation (especially with history of a break in the skin or insect bite), I treat this as a possible infection. Systemic cephalexin is a good choice for empiric therapy. I also swab any discharge for culture and sensitivity to guide therapy.

97

If there is a classic presentation of a focally tender point in the eyelid with overlying erythema, a hordeolum or acute chalazion is the likely diagnosis (Figure 22-1). My initial treatment includes aggressive warm compresses to promote spontaneous drainage of the lesion. If there is a plugged meibomian gland, the plug is removed at the slit lamp with a forceps or wooden end of a cotton-tipped applicator.[1] Antibiotics are seldom needed as secondary infection is rare. However, topical erythromycin ointment can be helpful for ocular surface comfort and treating underlying blepharitis and potential secondary infection. I occasionally prescribe systemic antibiotics for patients with severe inflammation resembling preseptal cellulitis. If there is obvious pointing of the lesion, you can promote drainage by unroofing it with the tip of an 18-gauge needle.

If a chalazion does not drain within a month or 2 and is no longer inflamed, it becomes chronic and is usually encapsulated. Hot soaks are usually ineffective at this point, and, if symptomatic, I recommend surgical incision and drainage.

Treatment of Chronic Chalazia

Chronic chalazia have been shown to respond to steroid injections. Triamcinolone 10-40 mg/mL can be injected from a posterior approach directly into the lesion. A total volume of 0.1 to 0.2 mL is sufficient.[2] I avoid injecting darker pigmented patients because hypopigmentation can occur with steroid injection. Lash loss is also a risk factor, and you need to counsel patients regarding this risk as well as the rare complication of intraocular embolization with steroid injections.

My preferred treatment for chronic chalazion is incision and drainage with curettage and direct excision of the capsule from a posterior approach. I inject the eyelid around the chalazion with 1.5 mL of 1% lidocaine with 1:100,000 epinephrine. Clamp the lid with a chalazion clamp with the ring-side touching the conjunctival side of the lid, and evert the lid. Be sure it is tight enough to stabilize the lid and help with hemostasis, but not so tight that it causes crush injury to the adjacent tarsus. Use a #11 scalpel blade to cut vertically along the superior part of the tarsus without cutting the full height of the tarsus to maintain lid stability. Vertical incisions will decrease the number of damaged tarsal glands as they run vertically within the tarsus. Yellowish-white granulomatous material will usually present itself. Use a chalazion curette to remove the granulomatous materiel (Figure 22-2). Use enough force to break up loculated areas, which may have developed with time. Then, using a 0.3 forceps or Bishop forceps, grasp the whitish capsule under the edge of the conjunctiva and dissect out as much of the capsule as possible (Figure 22-3). This will decrease the risk of recurrence of the chalazion. I use a battery-operated handheld cautery device for judicious hemostasis. Excessive cautery can cause lid notching and lash loss. Alternatively, apply antibiotics and a pressure patch for 10 to 15 minutes after the procedure for hemostasis.

If the chalazion appears unusual, recurs, or looks like asymmetric blepharitis, do a full-thickness biopsy using a small wedge resection and primary closure technique, and send the specimen to rule out a diagnosis of sebaceous cell carcinoma.

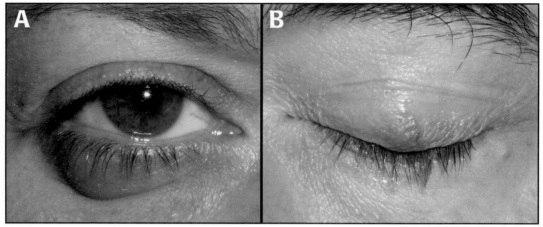

Figure 22-1. Acute (A) and chronic (B) chalazia.

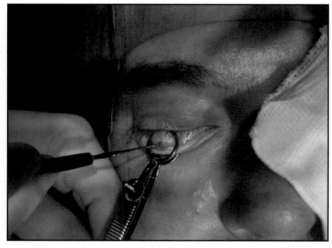

Figure 22-2. Chalazion clamp in place over chalazion with ring side facing conjunctiva and chalazion curette removing contents of chalazion.

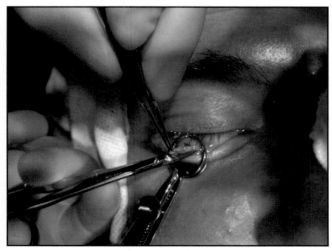

Figure 22-3. Excision of chalazion fibrous capsule after subconjunctival dissection.

Associated Findings

Blepharitis or meibomitis with or without accompanying acne rosacea is a common finding in patients with hordeola and chalazia, especially if the chalazia are multiple and recurrent. Carefully examine patients for these underlying diseases, and treat them accordingly. Ocular involvement can often precede classical cutaneous findings of rosacea.[3] Prescribe a regimen of warm soaks, lid scrubs, and erythromycin ointment at bedtime and flax seed oil capsules 4 times daily to treat the posterior blepharitis. In more severe cases, I also prescribe doxycycline 50 mg twice daily until the disease is under control, then maintain on a once-daily dose with the possibility of cycling on and off the oral medication every 3 to 4 months depending upon individual response.

References

1. Burkhart CG, Burkhart CN. Similar to acne vulgaris, bacteria may produce the biological glue that causes plugging of the meibomian gland leading to chalazia. *Clin Experiment Ophthalmol.* 2008;36(3):295.
2. Brown TM, Pandya VB, Masselos K, et al. A prospective randomized treatment study comparing three treatment options for chalazia: triamcinolone acetonide injections, incision and curettage and treatment with hot compresses: comment. *Clin Experiment Ophthalmol.* 2008;36(4):394-395.
3. Chamaillard M, Mortemousque B, Boralevi F, et al. Cutaneous and ocular signs of childhood rosacea. *Arch Dermatol.* 2008;144(2):167-171.

23

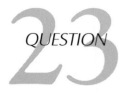

A 13-YEAR-OLD FEMALE IS COMPLAINING OF AN ENLARGING BROWN SPOT ON HER EYE. THE EXAM SHOWS A FLAT CONJUNCTIVAL PIGMENTED NEVUS THAT IS 3 MM IN DIAMETER SURROUNDED BY MILD CONJUNCTIVAL INJECTION. SHOULD I BE WORRIED ABOUT MALIGNANCY?

Frederick (Rick) W. Fraunfelder, MD
(co-authored with Michael A. Page, MD)

The differential diagnosis of pigmented conjunctival lesions includes congenital conjunctival freckles, melanocytosis, conjunctival nevi, racial melanosis, primary acquired melanosis (PAM), and malignant melanoma.[1] There are also many secondary causes of pigmented conjunctival lesions, such as drug-related pigment deposits and metabolic diseases leading to pigmented conjunctiva. Pigmented lesions of the ocular surface are relatively common and are typically benign. Because they can arise from a number of cell types and can be influenced by a variety of environmental factors, lesion characteristics and patient history are helpful in making the correct diagnosis.

Benign Conjunctival Nevus

The case presented here most likely represents a benign conjunctival nevus. The history and exam findings for our 13-year-old patient are most consistent with this diagnosis as conjunctival nevi typically appear in childhood as small, flat, circumscribed lesions near the limbus in the interpalpebral region (Figure 23-1). They are found less often at

Figure 23-1. Conjunctival nevus with cysts.

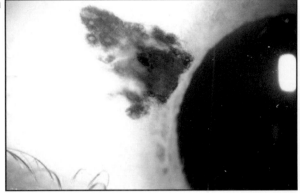

the caruncle or semilunar fold and rarely involve the palpebral conjunctiva or lid margin. They may or may not be pigmented, and they can vary from pink to yellow-tan to dark brown.

Incidence is 1.2:10 million people/year in all races. Conjunctival nevi are hamartomas and are described by their histological configuration as junctional, compound, or sub-epithelial.

Junctional nevi are located only within the epithelium and are rarely found except in children. They are difficult to distinguish histopathologically from PAM. Compound nevi are more common and involve both epithelium and subconjunctival connective tissue. Approximately 50% of these contain small epithelial inclusion cysts, which are lined by cuboidal cells and goblet cells. Sub-epithelial nevi are typically nonpigmented and often have a cobblestone appearance.

Before discussing management, it may be worthwhile to describe the other possibilities listed in the differential diagnosis.

Conjunctival Freckles

Ephelis, or conjunctival freckles, are flat brown patches typically found on the bulbar conjunctiva near the limbus. They are typically small and do not carry malignant potential. Ephelis are more common in darkly pigmented individuals and may arise in early childhood rather than at birth. Their pigmentation remains stable over time, and the surrounding conjunctiva is normal. Histologically, the conjunctival epithelium appears normal aside from a well-circumscribed area of hyperpigmented basal cells.

Ocular Melanocytosis

Ocular melanocytosis is another common congenital condition, occurring in 1/2500 individuals and found most typically in Black, Hispanic, and Asian groups. Typically unilateral and affecting the episclera, this condition presents with non-mobile slate-grey patches that are visible through normal conjunctiva. Iris and choroid may be involved, and many patients have ipsilateral dermal involvment in cranial nerve V distribution (oculodermal melanocytosis, or nevus of Ota). There is some risk of malignant

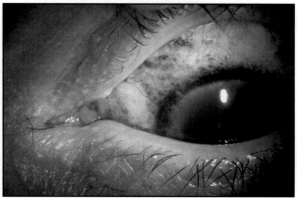

Figure 23-2. Diffuse primary acquired melanosis.

transformation, with the lifetime risk of uveal melanoma about 1 in 400. Secondary glaucoma occurs in 10% of affected eyes.

Benign Racial Melanosis

Benign melanosis, also known as racial melanosis, is a bilateral, diffuse, patchy increase in pigmentation of the bulbar conjunctiva. Typically found in middle-aged patients with dark skin, the incidence varies with racial groups: 92.5% in Blacks, 36% in Asians, 28% in Hispanics, and 4.9% in Caucasians. These lesions represent melanocytic hyperplasia, which may be triggered by sunlight exposure or other stimuli. Typically flat and affecting the perilimbal and interpalpebral bulbar conjunctiva, these lesions do not carry malignant potential.

Primary Acquired Melanosis

PAM typically affects white middle-aged patients and initially appears as flat, brown lesions of the conjunctival epithelium (Figure 23-2). These lesions are unilateral and may affect any part of the bulbar or palpebral conjunctiva. They may be analogous to lentigo maligna of the skin (also known as Hutchinson's freckle) and are therefore considered to be a premalignant condition. PAM is relatively common, affecting approximately 36% of Caucasian patients. Histology demonstrates a spectrum of epithelial involvement by abnormal melanocytes, ranging from mild increased pigmentation of the basal epithelium to formation of melanocytic nests to microinvasion of the substantia propria (signifying melanoma). PAM with atypia, a histologic description based upon biopsy, is a strong predictor for malignant transformation. Studies indicate that 33% to 46% of these lesions will progress to melanoma, within an average time of 2.5 years.

There are many other secondary causes of benign acquired melanosis. Melanin-like pigmentation of the conjunctiva may appear in patients on certain topical and systemic medications such as epinephrine ("adrenochrome deposits"), tetracycline, or silver-containing compounds. Trauma or chronic inflammation may induce migration of melanocytes or melanin-containing macrophages into the superficial conjunctiva and cause patchy pigmentation. Metabolic diseases such as ochronosis or hemachromatosis are potential causes, as are copper or iron-containing metallic foreign bodies.

Figure 23-3. Conjunctival malignant melanoma.

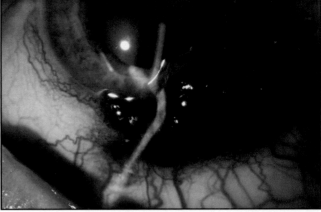

Malignant Melanoma

Malignant melanoma of the conjunctiva may arise from PAM, from acquired nevi, or de novo from normal conjunctiva. It is the second most common malignant neoplasm of the conjunctiva after squamous cell carcinoma. With a prevalence of 1:2 million among Caucasians, it is a relatively rare condition and is exceedingly rare in children or adolescents.[2] These lesions tend to grow in a nodular fashion and are highly vascularized, so they may bleed (Figure 23-3). They may invade the globe or orbit, though rates of metastasis are lower than that for cutaneous melanoma. Melanomas of the bulbar conjunctiva carry a better prognosis than those on the palpebral conjunctiva or caruncle. Occasionally, melanomas of the uvea may erode through the sclera and mimic a conjunctival lesion.

Management

Increased mucin production by the goblet cells contained in nevus cysts may cause abrupt but benign enlargement of the lesion. Inflammation can also induce an increase in nevus size, and a nevus may grow in a benign fashion with puberty or pregnancy (as in our case). Rapid growth of a pigmented lesion outside of these circumstances, increase in nodularity, bleeding, or involvement of the cornea or palpebral tissues are more concerning for risk of malignancy. A new lesion arising from an area of PAM is similarly concerning. In these cases, excisional biopsy ± cryotherapy is recommended.[3] If no concerning features are present and the lesion presents no cosmetic problem to the patient, then observation is warranted.

References

1. Shields CL, Dermirci H, Karatza E, Shields JA. Clinical survey of 1643 melanocytic and nonmelanocytic conjunctival tumors. *Ophthalmology.* 2004;111(9):1747-1754.
2. Jakobiec FA, Rini FJ, Fraunfelder FT, Brownstein S. Cryotherapy for conjunctival primary acquired melanosis and malignant melanoma. Experience with 62 cases. *Ophthalmology.* 1988;95(8):1058-1070.
3. Fraunfelder FW. Liquid nitrogen cryotherapy for surface eye disease (an AOS thesis). *Trans Am Ophthalmol Soc.* 2008;106:301-324.

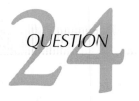

A 52-Year-Old Obese Male Comes to the Office Complaining of Pain and Irritation in the Right Eye. The Exam Shows Floppy Eyelids, 3+ Papillae in Upper Tarsal Conjunctiva, and Lash Ptosis. Does He Need Eyelid Surgery?

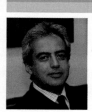

Reza Dana, MD, MSc, MPH

Floppy eyelid syndrome (FES) was first described in 1981,[1] exclusively in overweight men presenting with papillary conjunctivitis and floppy eyelids. It is now known that non-obese patients, women, and even children can develop FES, but the correlation remains highest with middle-aged obese men.

Symptoms

Symptoms in FES are generally nonspecific. Patients often complain of chronic irritation in one or both eyes with occasional or constant redness and/or mucus discharge.[2] Itching and chronic eye rubbing are also occasionally noted. Patients often present with a long history of using numerous topical medications/eye drops with little to no relief.

Signs

The cardinal clinical finding in FES is the easily everted upper eyelid. Even gentle lifting of the upper eyelid can lead to lid eversion (Figure 24-1). The lid often has a "rubbery" feel to it with abnormal thickness—the tarsus, rather than being rigid, is pliable and soft. Patients almost always have varying degrees of chronic papillary conjunctivitis that is unilateral or bilateral. Sometimes, lash ptosis, ectropion, or blepharoptosis are also seen. The most significant involvement in FES is corneal. This can range from focal punctate epitheliopathy (seen in nearly half of patients) to superficial neovascularization and scarring. Significant thinning, ulceration, and even perforation have also been reported, but these are rare. Up to 10% of FES patients may also have keratoconus. Eye rubbing, which is commonly seen in many keratoconus patients, is also seen in many FES patients, but it is not known if this is a cause or consequence of the eyelid pathology.

Histological and cytological studies, though rarely used or needed, can occasionally be helpful in confirming the diagnosis. Pathological examination of resection specimens from the tarsus shows rupture and loss of elastin fibers in the tarsus. Cytological evaluation of the ocular surface shows a nonspecific chronic inflammatory infiltrate in the conjunctival epithelium.[3]

Systemic Associations with FES

It is helpful to consider the various associations with FES, not only in consideration of the differential diagnosis (see below) but also in the overall management of the patients. The vast majority of patients with FES are obese with a significantly elevated body mass index (BMI). There is a strong association with obstructive sleep apnea, which itself is also associated with obesity. Only a minority of patients (~2% to 30%) with obstructive sleep apnea have FES, but nearly half of FES patients have sleep apnea—an important consideration in the management of these patients. Other co-morbidities seen in these patients are those commonly seen in obese patients, including systemic hypertension and hyperglycemia.

Pathogenesis

The exact pathogenesis of FES is unknown. Several theories have been proposed.[2] The most common relates FES to mechanical rubbing of the floppy eyelid on the pillow or sheets causing eyelid eversion and keratoconjunctivitis. This is supported by the association of FES with the side the patient sleeps on. Another theory proposes that pressure-induced ischemia and reperfusion leads to oxidative injury. Local "ischemia" or hypoperfusion may lead to elevated expression of matrix metalloprotease enzymes that degrade elastin and cause eyelid floppiness.

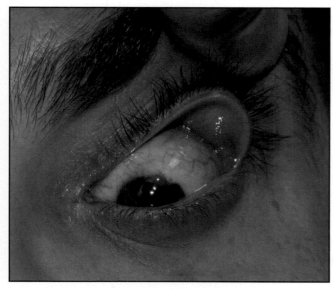

Figure 24-1. Clinical photograph demonstrating easy eversion of the upper eyelid in a patient with floppy eyelid syndrome. (Photo courtesy of Dr. Aaron Fay, Massachusetts Eye and Ear Infirmary, Boston, MA.)

Differential Diagnosis

Except for the floppy eyelids, none of the other findings are particularly specific. Chronic ocular irritation, redness, and mucus discharge are also frequently seen in dry eye syndromes, blepharitis, and allergy. For this reason, taking a good history and evaluation of non-ophthalmic findings, such as obesity and sleep apnea, can provide important clues to making the correct diagnosis.

Treatment Approaches

Like most other disorders, the most important parameter I consider for guiding me in therapy is the severity of the disease. The guidelines I use are as follows:

* In mild to moderate FES, without corneal thinning or extensive confluent epitheliopathy, conservative approaches often suffice. This involves (a) protecting the eyelid from spontaneous eversion and (b) protecting the cornea. Eyelid taping and/or application of a shield at bedtime can protect the eyelid from eversion in patients who can tolerate these approaches. Application of lubricating gels or ointments is protective of the cornea.

* Similarly, discontinuing chronic use of unneeded and potentially toxic medications such as antibiotics and anti-inflammatory treatments, including corticosteroids and nonsteroidal anti-inflammatory drugs (NSAIDs), is critical in protecting the cornea.

* However, in patients with severe FES or in those who are intolerant of shield application during sleep, surgical treatment is necessary. Surgical treatment typically consists of horizontal tightening procedures; many have been described to treat FES with a common recommended approach being a pentagonal eyelid wedge resection.

Surgical treatment usually is *not* directed at primarily correcting the ptosis, as this can improve with decreasing inflammation and lid-tightening procedures alone. Some oculoplastics specialists recommend that patients continue wearing a shield at night to prevent recurrence.

✳ It is critical to recall that obstructive sleep apnea is a serious and potentially fatal condition associated with cardiac disease and hypoxic organ damage; hence, it should be evaluated in FES patients, especially those who are obese. Good communication with the primary care physician is critical to ensure appropriate referral, sleep studies, and treatment of sleep apnea if present. Interestingly, it has been reported that treatment of sleep apnea may be associated with reversal of FES without any additional surgical intervention.[4]

References

1. Culbertson WW, Ostler HB. The floppy eyelid syndrome. *Am J Ophthalmol.* 1981;92(4):568-575.
2. Phamm TT, Perry JD. Floppy eyelid syndrome. *Curr Opin Ophthalmol.* 2007;18(5):430-433.
3. Medel R, Alonso T, Vela JI, Calatayud M, Bisbe L, Garcia-Arumi J. Conjunctival cytology in floppy eyelid syndrome: objective assessment of the outcome of surgery. *Br J Ophthalmol.* 2009;93(4):513-517.
4. McNab AA. Reversal of floppy eyelid syndrome with treatment of obstructive sleep apnoea. *Clin Exp Ophthalmol.* 2000;28(2):125-126.

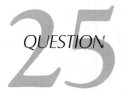

A 72-Year-Old Male Is Complaining of Decreased Vision. The Exam Shows Nuclear Cataract and Cortical Spoking. In the Area Above the Cortical Spokes, There Is a Pigmented Lesion of the Iris and Ectropion Uvea. Should I Arrange for Excision of the Lesion?

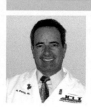

Henry Daniel Perry, MD

Pigmented lesions of the iris are relatively common.[1] Not infrequently, patients only notice an iris lesion after questioning by the ophthalmologist. By far, the most common lesion is the iris nevi. Most iris nevi tend to be stationary and non-progressive. However, they can occasionally affect the pupillary margin, angle, lens, or anterior chamber. Probably the most common pupillary change is ectropion iridis. Characteristically, ectropion iridis is associated with iris nevi near the pupillary margin. This pupillary sign may be interpreted as reflecting a malignant transformation. This is rarely the case. Many iris nevi may also be associated with a sector cortical cataract in the quadrant of the lesion. This type of change may remain stable for many years. The development of this type of cataract in the majority of cases also does not imply malignant transformation even if the cataract is progressive.

Differential Diagnosis

The other entities in the differential diagnosis of a pigmented lesion of the iris include iris melanocytoma, iris melanoma, iris nevus (Cogan-Reese) syndrome, iris cysts, and intraocular foreign bodies. Iris melanocytomas tend to be almost black in appearance and frequently undergo spontaneous necrosis. This necrotic change can lead to seeding cells and debris in the anterior chamber and trabecular meshwork and occasionally an ipsilateral glaucoma.[2]

Iris melanomas are usually greater than 3 mm in diameter and 1 mm in height. Any mass smaller than this would be most likely considered an iris nevus. Melanomas also tend to be more vascular with prominent feeding vessels. They are also invariably located in the lower half of the iris (Figure 25-1).

The iris nevus syndrome is characterized by multiple nevi that are actually areas of normal iris trapped and constricted by anomalous Descemet's membrane. This ectopic Descemet's membrane extends from the posterior cornea to envelope, constrict, and compress normal areas of the iris causing them to appear to be nevi. This entity is a variant of iridocorneal endothelial syndrome.

Iris cysts usually occur in younger patients and are more common in women than men. They are commonly found on routine evaluations when they displace the iris.

Intraocular foreign bodies may closely resemble iris tumors. Frequently, there is a history of trauma, but this fact may be overlooked due to the passage of time. Careful slit-lamp evaluation will frequently identify the site of entrance in the cornea. Metallic foreign bodies may oxidize and appear indistinguishable from an iris melanocytic lesion. Ultrasonography will clearly distinguish such lesions.[3] Other iris lesions such as leiomyoma, hemangioma, metastatic tumor, rhabdomyosarcoma, juvenile xanthogranuloma, tuberculosis, and sarcoidosis are all non-pigmented.

If an iris pigmented lesion extends into the angle and has been clearly documented to be growing or producing a secondary glaucoma that was unresponsive to medical therapy, an iridotrabeculectomy would be indicated (Figure 25-2). This type of biologic behavior is more characteristic of melanoma than iris nevi. The findings of an iris mass invading into the inferior angle with an unrelenting glaucoma and prominent vascularity would all point to the diagnosis of iris melanoma. Prominent vascularity alone, such as vessels that ramify throughout the lesion as a single finding in a mass 3 mm or larger, would also point toward malignancy.

What About Management?

If the diagnosis is iris nevi, cataract surgery alone may be performed without any iris surgery and would be the patient's best option. Even if the diagnosis is iris melanoma, the majority of cases may be handled by cataract surgery alone. The reasons for this reflect conclusions of experience from managing iris melanomas from several large studies. They all suggest that death from an iris melanoma is rare at worst and may never occur except in the rare instance of a diffuse melanoma of the iris where the mortality may reach 10% in 10 years.[4] Iris melanomas may be locally invasive and eventually lead to loss of the eye, but truly metastatic disease has not been clearly demonstrated in non-diffuse

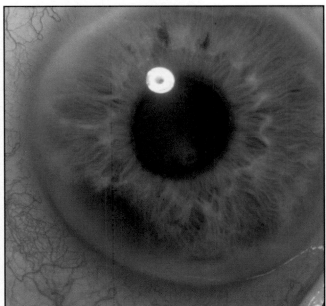

Figure 25-1. External photograph showing an inferior melanoma extending into the angle in a patient with secondary glaucoma.

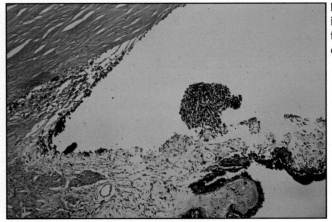

Figure 25-2. Histophotograph showing a melanoma of the iris seeding the angle in a patient whose glaucoma required enucleation.

iris melanomas. Therefore, I usually recommend a conservative approach. Slit-lamp photography is helpful in following these lesions, which, as a group, tend to be slow growing or stationary. I am careful to do a thorough retinal indirect examination and ultrasound studies to rule out ciliary body involvement, which would change the diagnosis to ciliary body melanoma necessitating a different management approach. I have recommended on occasion the excision of large melanocytic tumors that contact the cornea as well as the chamber angle. One such patient refused removal of her 6 mm iris mass at the time of phacoemulsification. Interestingly, 10 years later, the patient has maintained excellent vision, and the mass is relatively unchanged.

In summary, for the majority of cases of pigmented tumors of the iris, a conservative approach is recommended.[5] Should growth occur, look for signs of angle involvement, extrascleral extension, prominent vascularity, and glaucoma as reasons for concern.

References

1. Shields JA. *Diagnosis and Management of Intraocular Tumors*. St. Louis, MO: CV Mosby; 1983.
2. Shields JA, Shields CL, Eagle RC Jr. Melanocytoma (hyperpigmented magnocellular nevus) of the uveal tract: the 34th G. Victor Simpson lecture. *Retina*. 2007;27(6):730-739.
3. Nordlund JR, Robertson DM, Herman DC. Ultrasound biomicroscopy in management of malignant iris melanoma. *Arch Ophthalmol*. 2003;121(5):725-727.
4. Demirci H, Shields CL, Shields JA, Eagle RC Jr, Honavar SG. Diffuse iris melanoma: a report of 25 cases. *Ophthalmology*. 2002;109(8):1553-1560.
5. Conway RM, Chua WC, Qureshi C, Billson FA. Primary iris melanoma: diagnostic features and outcome of conservative surgical treatment. *Br J Ophthalmol*. 2001;85(7):848-854.

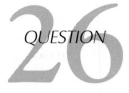

A YOUNG PATIENT WITH RECURRENT EPISODES OF THYGESON'S KERATITIS WANTS ME TO REFILL A PRESCRIPTION FOR TOPICAL CORTICOSTEROIDS THAT SHE USES INTERMITTENTLY AS NEEDED FOR DISCOMFORT. SHOULD I DO IT?

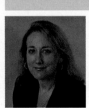

Jayne S. Weiss, MD

The steroid prescription should not be refilled unless there is confirmation of the diagnosis, determination that topical steroid is the optimal treatment for this patient, and arrangements for follow up of the patient have been made to confirm there are no steroid-related side effects.

How Is Thygeson's Diagnosed?

A complete dilated exam should be performed. Slit-lamp examination will reveal if the patient has the multiple characteristic whitish corneal intraepithelial deposits (Figure 26-1). The intraepithelial location of the deposits can be confirmed with fluorescein staining. The deposits cause elevation of the epithelium so these areas look more intensely blue than the surrounding epithelium—a characteristic called negative staining (Figure 26-2). The location and number of intraepithelial deposits vary with each attack. Dilated fundus exam will determine if the patient has developed any steroid-related complications such as cataract or glaucoma.

Figure 26-1. Slit-lamp photograph demonstrating 2 intraepithelial opacities in a patient with Thygeson's keratitis. (Photo courtesy of Christopher Rapuano, MD.)

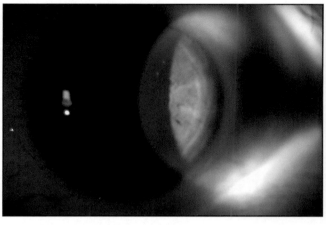

Figure 26-2. Slit-lamp photograph with fluorescein demonstrating staining of intraepithelial opacity. (Photo courtesy of Christopher Rapuano, MD.)

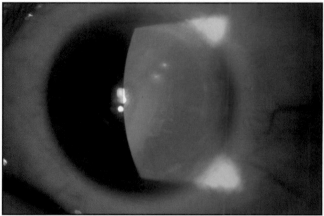

Unfortunately, the slit-lamp examination may be normal if the patient is presenting during the quiescent phase. So, history may provide the only clue to the diagnosis. Typically, patients will report attacks of ocular irritation, which may occur in one or the other eye. Symptoms may include burning, irritating, tearing, photophobia, and foreign body sensation. Frequently, many other ophthalmologists have been previously consulted because the attacks continue despite trials of different ocular medications. While the symptoms are non-specific, the recurrent episodes are characteristic.

An observational case series of 40 patients at Wills Eye Hospital with Thygeson's keratitis revealed a mean patient age of 28.7 years, and the most common presenting symptoms were photophobia, blurred vision, and irritation. Eighty-four percent of patients had bilateral disease. Almost 79% of patients without a history of decreased vision had visual acuity of 20/30 in both eyes or better, and 21% of patients had visual acuity between 20/40 and 20/50.[1]

If a new patient has no corneal signs of Thygeson's keratitis, I require more detailed history before I write a prescription for topical corticosteroids. I like to ask, "What doctor has been following you? When did you last see him or her? Can we get the old records?" Because of the multiple recurrences over years, patients may prefer to self-medicate and avoid doctor visits. A patient who checks in with doctors every few years only after they run out of the corticosteroid prescription refills may be at higher risk for steroid-related complications, such as cataract and glaucoma.

What Are the Treatment Options?

The mainstay of treatment of Thygeson's keratitis is topical steroids. I will often begin prednisolone acetate 1% 4 times a day until the deposits resolve and then perform a slow taper to avoid a rapid recurrence. The Wills series found that 97.5% of their patients were treated with topical steroids. It is imperative that these patients be told of the possible side effects of topical steroids including elevated intraocular pressure and cataract formation, and it is imperative that the physician document in the medical record that this conversation took place. I have seen patients who have been able to receive multiple steroid drop refills without seeing the ophthalmologist and persisted in treating their own recurrences, only to return to the ophthalmologist years later with steroid-related cataract or glaucoma.

Topical cyclosporine (0.5% or 2%) has been used in some cases to successfully treat Thygeson's keratitis, specifically if there is contraindication to topical steroid or concern about potential side effects.[2]

While both PRK and LASIK have been reported in these patients, intraepithelial deposits have been reported to recur after either procedure.[3]

Supportive therapy with artificial tears is often used, but this does not change the course or resolve the deposits. Likewise, bandage contact lenses can cover up the deposits and relieve the foreign body sensation but will not change the course of the disease.

What Is the Natural Course and Duration of Disease?

In the Wills series, the patients followed for more than 1 year had an average duration of the disease of 11.1 years. Patients may have multiple recurrences in either eye. The challenge of dosing topical steroid or cyclosporine therapy is determining how slow a medication taper should be in order to avoid a rapid recurrence of the keratitis. Some patients require weeks of therapy. With successful treatment, frequency of recurrences varies among individual patients.

References

1. Nagra PK, Rapuano CJ, Cohen EJ, Laibson PR. Thygeson's superficial punctate keratitis: ten years' experience. *Ophthalmology.* 2004;111(1):34-37.
2. Reinhard T, Sundmacher R. Topical cyclosporine A in Thygeson's superficial punctate keratitis. *Graefes Arch Clin Exp Ophthalmol.* 1999;237(2):109-112.
3. Netto MV, Chalita MR, Krueger RR. Thygeson's superficial punctate keratitis: Recurrence after laser in situ keratomileusis. *Am J Ophthalmol.* 2004;138(3):507-508.

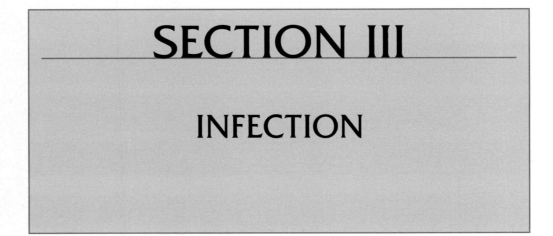

SECTION III

INFECTION

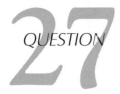

A PATIENT PRESENTS WITH CORNEAL ULCER. WHAT WORK-UP AND TREATMENT WOULD YOU RECOMMEND?

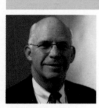

John W. Cowden, MD

Prashant Garg, MD

Martin Filipec, MD, PhD

Note: This particular question is unique in this book as there is one question and 3 different responses. We did this because there can be different approaches to an apparent corneal ulcer based on the location and available antibiotics. This book is intended to be helpful to doctors around the world. We chose an author from the Midwestern United States, India, and Europe.

By John W. Cowden, MD

Ophthalmic examination of the patient who presents with a corneal ulcer (Figure 27-1) begins with a detailed history of the onset, duration, prior ocular diseases or trauma, ocular medications, use of contact lenses and solutions, and outdoor activities such as gardening or farming. Symptoms of pain and decreased vision, redness, and type of discharge are also noted. Slit-lamp examination is done to determine the ulcer's location; morphology; and the severity of edema, infiltrates, and thinning (Figure 27-2). Anterior chamber reaction is assessed, noting cells, flare, keratic precipitates, and hypopyon. Corneal sensation is tested using a wisp of cotton. Fluorescein is then instilled to reveal the extent of the epithelial defect. A drawing of the corneal ulcer is made, including a depiction of the location, degree of stromal infiltrate, the size of the epithelial defect, and morphology.

Identification

A corneal scraping for smears and cultures is required whenever the epithelium is not intact.[1] Because a corneal ulcer often yields scant material for a specimen, I prefer to obtain the smears and apply the scrapings directly onto the culture media. A gram stain for bacteria, Giemsa stain, and a Gridley modified PAS stain for fungus are ordered. Cultures are plated on blood agar, chocolate agar, and Sabouraud's media, along with liquid media of thioglycolate broth or beef heart infusion. Viral transport media is inoculated. I also collect a separate culturette for polymerase chain reaction (PCR) for herpes simplex virus (HSV), if it is suspected. If acanthamoeba or chronic keratitis is suspected, an *E. coli* overlay plate for acanthamoeba is requested from the laboratory.

Culture specimens should be obtained when the patient is initially seen, before treatment begins. The specimen is obtained from the site of major inflammatory activity, plated immediately, and inoculated into non-dehydrated liquid media. Follow-up personal contact with the laboratory is essential.

Treatment

Small peripheral non-staining corneal infiltrates with minimal anterior chamber reaction are generally treated with moxifloxacin (Vigamox) or gatifloxacin (Zymar), one drop every 2 to 4 hours. If moderate infection is present, the topical fluoroquinolone should be administered every hour until improvement occurs. Then, the dose is reduced. Therapy continues until the ulcer is completely healed, which often takes several weeks.

The situation commonly arises in which the referring doctor initiated topical antibiotics for a corneal ulcer but no improvement occurs. In such cases, fortified vancomycin and fortified tobramycin are instituted, every hour around the clock for the first 2 to 3 days (Table 27-1).[2] If a fluoroquinolone was the initial agent, it can be continued every 2 hours while awake. For severe ulcers, particularly gram-negative ulcers, subconjunctival gentamicin or tobramycin, 40 mg/mL, is given daily for 3 days. A cycloplegic agent is administered until the anterior chamber reaction resolves. Frequent follow-up examinations are required until improvement is seen. Outpatient management is possible in the reliable patient who understands the importance of administering the drops each hour during the day and every 1 to 2 hours at night and will keep the daily follow-up

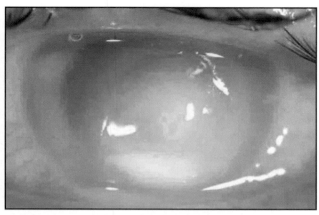

Figure 27-1. Corneal ulcer with a large central ring infiltrate and hypopyon.

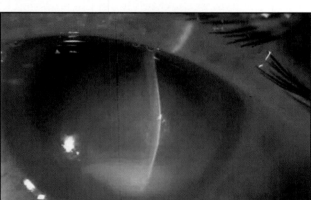

Figure 27-2. Slit-lamp appearance of a corneal ulcer of 3 days' duration caused by *Pseudomonas aeruginosa.*

<u>Table 27-1</u>

Preparation of Different Types of Fortified Antibiotics for the Treatment of Corneal Ulcers

Fortified antibiotic	*Instructions for preparation*
Gentamicin or tobramycin, 14 mg/mL	Add 2 mL of parenteral antibiotic (40 mg/mL) to a 5-mL bottle of gentamicin or tobramycin, 3 mg/mL.
Vancomycin, 50 mg/mL	Withdraw 2 mL of balanced salt solution (BSS) or an artificial tear solution from a 10-mL bottle, and inject it into the vial of powdered vancomycin, 500 mg. When in solution, withdraw the entire volume, and inject back into the bottle that contains 8 mL of BSS or artificial tears.
Cefazolin, 50 mg/mL	Add 10 mL of BSS or artificial tears to 500 mg of cefazolin dry powder to form a 10-mL solution of cefazolin, 50 mg/mL, which is injected into a sterile eye drop bottle.

Adapted from Chandler JW, Sugar J, Edelhauser HF. External diseases: cornea, conjunctiva, sclera, eyelids, lacrimal system. In: Podos SM, Yanoff M, eds. *Textbook of Ophthalmology,* Vol 8. London, UK: Mosby; 1994:11.8.

appointments. If the patient is unreliable or cannot administer the drops, hospitalization is required. The patient is examined daily until improvement is noted. Antibiotic therapy is then decreased to every 2 hours during the daytime and every 4 hours at night. Visit intervals can be extended to every 2 to 4 days.

If cultures are negative, no response occurs, or the condition is progressing, antibiotic therapy is discontinued overnight. Cultures and PCR for HSV are repeated the next day and a biopsy is done for fungal or acanthamoeba keratitis. The cornea should also be examined using the confocal microscope to look for acanthamoeba cysts.

The recent outbreaks of fusarium and acanthamoeba keratitis demand special consideration when the patient is a contact lens wearer.[3] Use of extended wear contacts and a history of swimming in a lake or using a hot tub increase the likelihood of amoebic keratitis.

The appropriate treatment for fungal keratitis is either natamycin (Natacyn) or amphotericin B every 1 to 2 hours around the clock. In addition, the overlying epithelium should be debrided daily and oral fluconazole or ketoconazole should be instituted 100 to 200 mg each day after the loading dose. If acanthamoeba is suspected or diagnosed, 1 drop of propamidine (Brolene) should be given every 2 hours, along with polyhexamethylene biguanide (Baquacil) or chlorhexidine hourly. Hourly Neosporin drops are also effective. Treatment must continue for at least 3 months after the inflammation has resolved. Often, up to 1 year is required. A mixed infection occasionally complicates the situation.[4] If new symptoms occur or the condition worsens, cultures are repeated and therapy is adjusted appropriately. Rarely, keratoplasty is required to save the eye. (The treatment of HSV keratitis is discussed in Question 34.)

Adjunctive therapy to reduce corneal scarring and heal persistent epithelial defects can be initiated once the infection is controlled and healing has commenced. Cautiously, I use prednisolone acetate (Pred Forte) 4 times daily (or less frequently). A bandage soft contact lens can be used to protect the cornea and promote healing. An amniotic membrane graft on a ring (ProKera) may be beneficial when a bandage soft contact lens is not helping to heal the epithelial defect.

The Key to Better Outcomes

Identifying the pathogen is extremely important. However, the pathogen often cannot be identified because antibiotics were used preceding cultures. The choice of an effective antibiotic used frequently and long enough usually eradicates the infection. Poor outcomes usually can be averted with appropriate, timely action.

References

1. Cohen EJ, Rapuano CJ. Bacteria keratitis, fungal keratitis, Acanthamoeba, herpes simplex virus, herpes zoster virus. In Kunimoto DY, Kanitkar KD, Maker MS, Friedberg MA, Rapuano CJ, eds. *The Wills Eye Manual: Office and Emergency Room Diagnosis and Treatment of Eye Disease*. 4th ed. Philadelphia, PA: Lippincott Williams & Wilkins. 2004:52-65.
2. Chandler JW, Sugar J, Edelhauser HF, eds. External diseases: cornea, conjunctiva, sclera, eyelids, lacrimal system. In: Podos SM, Yanoff M, eds. *Textbook of Ophthalmology*, Vol 8. London, England: Mosby. 1994:11.8.
3. Por YM, Mehta JS, Chua JL, et al. Acanthamoeba keratitis associated with contact lens wear in Singapore. *Am J Ophthlamol*. 2009;148(1):7-12.
4. Tu EY, Joslin CE, Nijm LM, Feder RS, Jain S, Shoff ME. Polymicrobial keratitis: acanthamoeba and infectious crystalline keratopathy. *Am J Ophthalmol*. 2009;148(1):13-19.

By Prashant Garg, MD

A corneal ulcer is characterized by an epitelial defect associated with underlying stromal infiltrate (Figure 27-3). Because it can be caused by a variety of infective and non-infective conditions, patients with ulcerative keratitis present both a diagnostic and therapeutic challenge to ophthalmologists. A systematic approach can help ophthalmologists better manage this condition.

Diagnosis

A detailed history and thorough clinical examination using the slit-lamp biomicroscope are important steps in the diagnosis of corneal ulcer. Pay attention to mode of onset of symptoms, duration, and rate of progression. If the patient has been treated elsewhere, note the details of the treatment and the response. If the patient wears contact lenses, it is important to know about the type of lenses (rigid gas-permeable [RGP] lenses or soft lenses), the wearing schedule, especially if the patient sleeps wearing lenses, and cleaning regimens including information on care of lens case. Inquire about any systemic illness, duration of the disease, and the treatment. This is important because systemic diseases such as rheumatoid arthritis and other collagen vascular diseases can cause ulcerative keratitis. Similarly, acne rosacea and other dermatological conditions can also produce sterile ulcerative keratitis.[1]

While you elicit history, pay attention to structures around the eyes. This will help you rule out disorders such as herpes zoster, acne rosacea, proptosis, and exposure keratitis or lagophthalmos.

Perform a thorough systematic slit-lamp examination with special attention to lids, including eyelashes, intermarginal strip and posterior lid margin, lacrimal sac, tear film, conjunctiva, sclera, cornea, anterior chamber, pupil, and posterior segment. While examining the cornea, note the location of the ulcer, size of epithelial defect and infiltrate, nature of the infiltrate and the character of the edge, depth of stromal involvement, and associated thinning or perforation. Examine the surrounding cornea for evidence of satellite lesions, immune rings, or radial keratoneuritis. Look for evidence of limbal or scleral involvement.

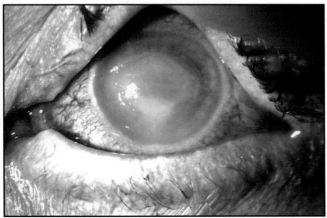

Figure 27-3. Corneal ulcer.

Try to document all findings in a schematic diagram as shown in Figure 27-4. This will help you properly analyze all of the clinical signs and assess the response to therapy during follow-up visits.

Although clinical signs may be insufficient to confirm infection, to be safe, a break in the continuity of the epithelium associated with underlying stromal suppuration should be considered infectious unless proven otherwise. While viral infections are the leading cause of corneal ulcer in developed nations, bacteria, fungi, and *acanthamoeba* all can invade the cornea to cause suppurative keratitis. A good practical approach to arriving at a diagnosis can be by looking at rate of progression and nature of infiltration (Table 27-2).

Some of the characteristic clinical pictures of infection by various organisms are shown in Figures 27-5 through 27-7.

Figure 27-4. Schematic documentation of a case of corneal ulcer.

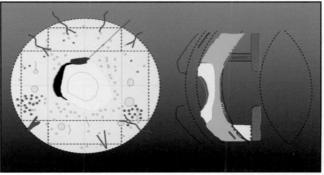

Table 27-2
Differential Diagnosis of Microbial Keratitis

Slowly progressive localized infiltrate bacteria:	Rapidly progressive diffuse suppurative infiltrate bacteria:
a) Gram positive	a) Gram positive
i) *Staphylococcus epidermidis*	i) *Staphylococcus aureus*
ii) α-hemolytic streptococci	ii) *Streptococcus pneumoniae*
iii) Actinomycetales	iii) ß-hemolytic streptococci
• *Actinomyces*	b) Gram negative
• *Nocardia*	i) *Pseudomonas*
• *Mycobacterium*	ii) *Enterobacteriaceae*
b) Gram negative	c) Mixed infection
i) Moraxella	d) Drug toxicity
ii) Serratia	

Fungi:
   a) Filamentous fungi (*Fusarium, Aspergillus,* Dematiaceous)
   b) Yeast (*Candida*)

Protozoa:
   a) *Acanthamoeba*
   b) Microsporidia

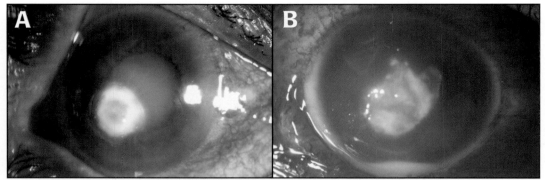

Figure 27-5. Corneal ulcer caused by gram-positive bacteria *S. pneumoniae* (A) and gram-negative bacteria *Pseudomonas aeruginosa* (B).

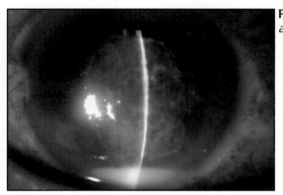

Figure 27-6. Corneal ulcer caused by *Nocardia asteroids.*

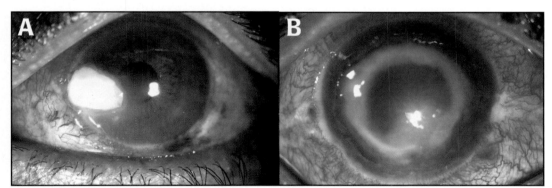

Figure 27-7. Corneal ulcer caused by filamentous fungi (A) and acanthamoeba (B).

It is important to remember that the clinical appearance of suppurative keratitis depends on many variables, and it is often difficult to arrive at an etiological diagnosis based entirely on slit-lamp examination.[2] Laboratory investigations are therefore required if the causative organism is to be identified. It consists of corneal scraping using #15 surgical blade or Kimura's spatula and inoculating it on various culture media that promote the growth of bacteria, fungi, and parasites as shown in Figure 27-8. The initial management is based on smear examination.

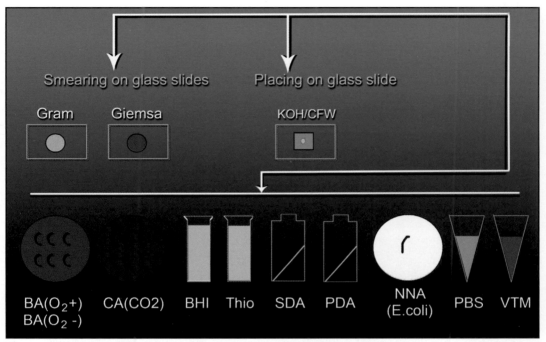

Figure 27-8. Schematic diagram of microbiology workup in corneal ulcer.

Management

Because facilities for detailed microbiology work-up may not be available to many ophthalmologists, bacteria cause a significant percentage of suppurative keratitis cases, and most antibacterial drugs are bactericidal, a practical approach could be used to perform laboratory work-up only in cases with severe keratitis (cases with corneal infiltrates more than 6 mm in size) or cases that show unusual clinical features.[3] In other cases, the following approaches can be adopted:

* Non-severe keratitis (infiltrates less than 2 mm in size) and no clinical signs of fungal or acanthamoeba infection: Treat empirically with broad-spectrum antibacterial therapy. Treatment can be started with one of the commercially available fourth-generation fluoroquinolones.

* Keratitis with infiltrates that are between 2 and 5 mm and no clinical signs of fungal or acanthamoeba infection: Treat with either fourth-generation fluoroquinolones or a combination of fortified cefazolin (5%) and ciprofloxacin 0.3%.

* Non-severe keratitis (infiltrate size less than 5 mm) with clinical evidence of fungal or acanthamoeba infection and in geographical locations where such infections are common: Perform corneal scrapings and examine the material under light microscope using 10% potassium hydroxide. Treatment with antifungal and anti-acanthamoeba drugs must be started only if smear is positive for these agents.

All antimicrobial drugs must be instilled frequently in the initial phase. All cases of severe keratitis must undergo inpatient treatment, while other cases can undergo outpatient treatment. However, we must review these cases almost every day for the first 3 to 4 days.

In addition to antimicrobial drugs, prescribe one of the cycloplegic agents and a systemic analgesic (if the patient has pain). Anti-glaucoma drugs are necessary only if intraocular pressure is high.

In addition to antimicrobial therapy, one must treat associated conditions that result in persistence or progression of ulcerative keratitis, such as conjunctival foreign body, lagophthalmos, meibomitis, dacryocystitis, or drug toxicity.

Treatment Adjustment

The modification of treatment is based on clinical response and culture results.

* If the patient is responding to initial therapy, reduce the frequency of instillation so as to maintain therapeutic corneal concentrations of the drugs.

* If the patient is not responding to initial therapy and microbiology work-up was not performed, perform a detailed microbiology work-up or refer the patient to centers where such facilities exist.

* If the patient is not responding and microbiology work-up was performed, review the results of the culture and antimicrobial susceptibility and modify therapy accordingly. Repeat the microbiology test or perform corneal biopsy if the tests are negative. In vivo confocal microscopy can be useful in patients with suspected fungal or acanthamoeba keratitis.[4]

All patients with advanced disease or failed medical treatment will require surgical treatment in the form of full-thickness penetrating or lamellar keratoplasty.[5]

The patient presented in this chapter has a large central corneal ulcer associated with inflammation of the lid margin. Because the infiltrate size is more than 6 mm, we must perform corneal scrapings in this case. Initial treatment must be based on results of microscopic examination of smears. In addition to antimicrobial therapy, this patient will require treatment of lid inflammation.

References

1. Sadowsky AE. Dermatological disorders. In Krachmer JH, Mannis MJ, Holland EJ. *Cornea*. St Louis, MO: Mosby. 1997:989-1002.
2. Thomas PA, Leck AK, Myatt M. Characteristic clinical features as an aid to the diagnosis of suppurative keratitis caused by filamentous fungi. *Br J Ophthalmol*. 2005;89(12):1554-1558.
3. McLeod SD, DeBacker CM, Viana MA. Differential care of corneal ulcers in the community based on apparent severity. *Ophthalmology*. 1996;103(3):479-484.
4. Kanavi MR, Javadi M, Yazdani S, Mirdehghanm S. Sensitivity and specificity of confocal scan in the diagnosis of infectious keratitis. *Cornea*. 2007;26(7):782-786.
5. Anshu A, Parthasarathy A, Mehta JS, Htoon HM, Tan DT. Outcomes of therapeutic deep lamellar keratoplasty and penetrating keratoplasty for advanced infectious keratitis: a comparative study. *Ophthalmology*. 2009;116(4):615-623.

BY MARTIN FILIPEC, MD, PhD

The slit-lamp photograph of this patient's cornea shows corneal epithelial defect, stromal infiltration, and hypopyon. This presentation (see Figure 27-3) is highly suspicious of infectious etiology, but it does not appear to have typical characteristics of any particular microorganism. Therefore, my differential would be broad and include bacteria, fungus, and acanthamoeba. The likelihood of viral etiology is very low in the presence of hypopyon, but it could be seen, particularly in an immunocompromised patient.

History

First, I take a detailed history that can increase the suspicion of a certain pathogen. Past medical history is focused on systemic diseases (diabetes mellitus, connective tissue diseases, vasculitic and infectious diseases, malignancy, use of immunosuppressive drugs, or presence of an immunocompromised condition) and ocular conditions (dry eye, recurrent erosion syndrome, herpetic infection, neurotrophic keratitis) predisposing the patient to infectious keratitis. I ask about the history of contact lens wear and, if present, the type of contact lenses and contact lens solution used, compliance with care for contact lenses, and exposure to swim water.

Examination

External exam is focused on signs of trauma or inflammation of eyelids and bulbar and tarsal conjunctiva. Slit-lamp examination is focused on presence or absence of epithelial defect; presence, location, and nature (solitary or satellite, epithelial or stromal) of infiltrate(s); presence or absence of stromal ulceration; necrosis; stromal thinning; Descemetocele impending; or present corneal perforation.

I always like to make the exact color drawing of the cornea along with slit-lamp photography. This helps a lot during the follow-up period, particularly when doubts about progression rise. Next is the examination of corneal sensation in both eyes. Marked asymmetry between the 2 eyes is highly suspicious of herpetic eye disease. In case the patient is a contact lens wearer, acanthamoeba must be considered in the differential diagnosis. This diagnosis is supported by findings of radial perineuritis and ring-shaped infiltrates. Extreme photophobia and pain are common symptoms of acanthamoeba keratitis, but they do not need to be present. One should bear in mind that 7% of acanthamoeba keratitis is not associated with contact lens wear.[1]

Work-Up

Next, corneal scraping for Gram stain, cultures, and sensitivities is performed. It is preferable to perform scraping without use of topical anaesthesia. If necessary, 1 drop of proparacaine hydrochloride 0.5% is used. Scraping from the ulcer is most important. I am usually not taking cultures from the eyelids and conjunctiva because their value is doubtful. I first clean the surface of the ulcer with the swab, and then I scrape the base and rim of the ulcer several times using a round knife or large needle. Harvested tissue from the cornea is collected by moistened Dacron swabs and inoculated in the form of C streaks to blood, chocolate, and Sabouraud's agar plates and into chopped meat broth (Table 27-3). One scraping is used for polymerase chain reaction for herpes simplex virus. Then, a smear is placed on 2 glass slides, which are then stuck together and sent to the laboratory for Gram and Blankophor (Bayer, Leverkusen, Germany) staining. If acanthamoeba etiology is suspected, I would ask for fresh mount light microscopy and staining of the smear with trichrome. I would also ask to culture scrapings, contact lens, and contact lens storage medium from the case (if available) on 1.5% non-nutrient agar plates seeded with heat-inactivated suspension of Escherichia coli (see Table 27-3). All media should stay at room temperature for 30 minutes after removal from the refrigerator to prevent the low temperature from interfering with the ability of microorganisms to grow. Stable room temperature must also be provided during the transport of the media to the laboratory[2] (Table 27-4).

Treatment

In the case of large central keratitis, I would start the initial treatment with topical antibiotics using fortified Tobramycin (14 mg/mL) and fortified cephazolin (50 mg/mL) alternating every 5 minutes during the first hour and then every hour around the clock. The nocturnal use of drops can be discontinued after 48 hours of therapy. For dilation and cycloplegia, I use homatropine 4% drops twice a day. The patient is asked to return for examination every other day during the first week and then according to the response. The therapy should be changed any time after the laboratory results show anything other than bacterial etiology that is sensitive to the antibiotics. In such cases, the specific therapy must be introduced. One could use ofloxacin 4 times a day as prophylaxis of secondary bacterial infection if antifungal, anti-amoeba, or antiviral agents are used. If bacteria are found as causative pathogens and there is no improvement within 4 to 5 days or the inflammation is getting worse, the therapy should then be changed according to the result of cultures and sensitivity. It is not common, but one should always think about a possibility of 2 concomitant causative infectious agents. Sometimes, the eye irritation can be caused by eye drop toxicity, and, in such cases, the frequency of administration should be tapered and/or changed. After fungal and herpetic etiology is ruled out and the infection is under control, it is possible to use topical corticosteroids to reduce the scar formation. I start using prednisolone acetate 1% 2 to 3 times a day and not earlier than 1 week after antibacterial treatment was introduced. One should bear in mind that corticosteroids are acting as a local immunosuppressive by preventing migration of neutrophils and by decreasing opsonisation, both of which can promote infection.[3] This is why corticosteroids should be used only when there is high certainty that the infection was eliminated. If the therapy is not successful and inflammation is progressing, I would stop the therapy for 24 to 48 hours and start again from the beginning with new laboratory examination and reconsideration of the diagnosis.

Table 27-3

Methods Used in Laboratory Diagnosis of Infectious Keratitis

Smears	Gram stain	Bacteria
	Blankophor	Fungi
	Fresh mount, trichrome	Acanthamoeba
Media	Blood agar	Most bacteria, yeast, fungi
	Chocolate agar	Most bacteria, Haemophilus, Neisseria, Moraxella
	Chopped meat broth	Aerobic and anaerobic bacteria
	Sabouraud's agar	Most fungi and yeast
	1.5% non-nutrient agar	Acanthamoeba
Polymerase chain reaction		Herpes simplex virus

Table 27-4

Potential Pitfalls During the Process of Laboratory Diagnosis

Scrapes and swabs	Only superficial debris on the surface of ulcer are taken Contamination Cotton swabs are inappropriate
Media	Old, inappropriate, or cold plates are used. The plates should stay 30 minutes at room temperature
Transport	Culture media are not kept room temperature during the transport
Interpretation of the result	Overestimation of nonpathogenic organisms and nonsignificant number of organisms

References

1. Radford CF, Lehman OJ, Dart JK. Acanthamoeba keratitis: multicentre survey in England 1992-6. *Br J Ophthalmol.* 1998;82(12):1387-1392.
2. BenEzra D. *Ocular Surface Inflammation: Guidelines for Diagnosis and Treatment.* Panama: Highlights of Ophthalmology International; 2003.
3. O'Brien TP. Bacterial keratitis. In: Foster CS, Azar DT, Dohlman CH, eds. *Smolin and Thoft's The Cornea: Scientific Foundations and Clinical Practice.* 4th ed. Philadelphia, PA: Lippincott Williams & Wilkins; 2005:235-288.

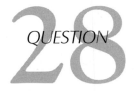

I HAVE A GENERAL OPHTHALMOLOGY PRACTICE IN A REMOTE AREA. WHEN SHOULD I CONSIDER DOING CORNEAL CULTURES?

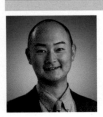

Francis S. Mah, MD

Bacterial colonization of the eyelid and conjunctiva is normal and helps reduce opportunities for pathogenic strains from gaining a foothold. Host defense mechanisms can be overcome, however, and lead to serious ocular morbidity if not treated properly. Although the clinical manifestations of corneal infections, such as history and exam, may be characteristic of certain pathogens, further laboratory evaluation with smears, cultures, and antibiotic susceptibility testing provide a definitive diagnosis and more focused treatment after empirical therapy has been initiated. However, in the current environment of cost-conscious health care in the world of excellent empiric therapies with clinically proven results, the question remains: When is laboratory evaluation by culture recommended for the practicing clinician?

Corneal Cultures and Smears

Routine culture of corneal infections (Figure 28-1) is not the usual practice in the community because almost all cases of keratitis resolve with empiric therapy.[1,2] However, smears and cultures are recommended in certain cases:

* A corneal infiltrate that is large (typically 2 mm or larger) and extends to the middle to deep stroma (ie, has stromal melting)

* A case that is chronic in nature or unresponsive to broad-spectrum antibiotic therapy

Figure 28-1. Less than 2 mm, peripheral corneal ulcer. May culture or treat empirically.

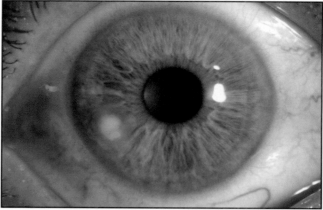

* A case with atypical clinical features suggestive of fungal, amoebic, or mycobacterial keratitis

* An unusual history (eg, trauma with vegetable matter) or using a hot tub while wearing contact lenses

* A sight-threatening or severe keratitis[3]

The hypopyon that occurs in eyes with severe bacterial keratitis is usually sterile, and aqueous or vitreous taps should not be performed due to possible intracameral introduction of the pathogen, unless there is a high suspicion of microbial endophthalmitis, such as following an intraocular surgery, perforating trauma, or sepsis.

A culture is a means of identifying the causative organism(s) and the only means of determining sensitivity to antibiotics. Cultures are helpful to guide modification of therapy in patients with a poor clinical response to treatment and to decrease toxicity by eliminating unnecessary medications. Corneal material is obtained by instilling a topical anesthetic agent. Topical anesthesia with proparacaine hydrochloride is preferred because it has fewer antibacterial properties than other topical anesthetics.[4] In addition, culture yield may be improved by avoiding anesthetics with preservatives.[5] A heat-sterilized platinum (Kimura) spatula, blade, jeweler's forceps, or other similar sterile instrument is used to obtain scrapings of material from the advancing borders of the infected area of the cornea as well as the base of the ulcer while carefully avoiding contamination from the lids and lashes. Obtaining only purulent material usually results in inadequate yield. Organisms such as *Streptococcus pneumoniae* are more readily recovered from the ulcer edge, while other organisms such as *Moraxella* are recovered from the base.[6] A thiol or thioglycolate broth-moistened Dacron/calcium alginate or sterile cotton swab may also be used to obtain material. It is important to remember that a wooden-stemmed swab is not optimal as it is an organic substance and, therefore, may produce a false-negative culture result. Culturing is most easily performed with slit-lamp magnification. The scrapings are inoculated onto solid media (blood, chocolate, mannitol, Sabouraud's agar) by streaking a row of Cs onto its surface. If a clinician were to choose only one medium to stock in the clinic, blood would be the recommended media of choice. New material is recovered for each row. Corneal scrapings for culture should be inoculated directly onto appropriate culture media in order to maximize culture yield.[7] If this is not feasible, specimens should be placed in transport media.[8,9] Cultures of the conjunctival cul-de-sac, lids and lashes, contact lenses, lens case, and solution may provide additional information to guide therapy. In eyes treated empirically without first obtaining cultures in which the clinical response is poor, obtaining cultures then may be helpful, although a delay in pathogen recovery may occur.[1,10] If the cultures are negative, the ophthalmologist may consider stopping antibiotic treatment for 12 to 24 hours and then re-culturing.

Microbial pathogens may also be categorized by examining stained smears of corneal scrapings.[11] This may increase the yield of identification of pathogen, especially if the patient is on antibacterial therapy. The material for smear is applied to clean glass microscope slides in an even, thin layer for Gram and Giemsa stains. Special stains include Ziehl-Neelsen acid-fast stain for *Mycobacterium*, *Actinomyces*, and *Nocardia*. Acridine orange is a fluorescent dye that may be helpful in identifying bacteria when yields are low, but this stain does not yield classification information that Gram's stain provides. Polymerase chain reaction (PCR) and immunodiagnostic techniques may be useful but are not currently widely available.[12,13]

When Is Biopsy Indicated and How Should It Be Done?

Corneal biopsy may be indicated if there has been a lack of response to treatment or if cultures have been negative on more than one occasion and the clinical picture continues to strongly suggest an infectious process. It may also be indicated if the infiltrate is located in the mid or deep stroma with overlying uninvolved tissue.[14,15] In a cooperative patient, corneal biopsy may be performed while at the slit-lamp biomicroscope or operating microscope. Using topical anesthesia, a small trephine (eg, 2-mm to 3-mm dermatic punch) or blade is used to excise a small piece of stromal tissue, which is large enough to allow bisection so that one portion can be sent for culture and the other for histopathology.[16] An option for a deep corneal abscess may be the use of a suture that can be passed through the abscess without disturbing the overlying intact corneal epithelium and stroma. A 7-0 or 8-0 vicryl or silk suture can be passed through the abscess. The choice of silk or vicryl is preferred because the pathogen may attach to the fibers of the suture. The suture is then cultured. Another option in cases of a deep corneal abscess with overlying clear cornea is to take the biopsy from below a lamellar flap, which can be created either manually or mechanically. An additional set of smears and cultures can be obtained from the deep stroma after the biopsy is performed.[16]

Summary

Although routine culturing of corneal infections is no longer the norm among practicing clinicians, it is the gold standard in identifying the etiology of keratitis pathogens. When used properly, judiciously, and in a timely fashion, it can be the sight-saving maneuver in the case of a difficult vision-devastating corneal infection.

References

1. McDonnell PJ, Nobe J, Gauderman WJ, Lee P, Aiello A, Trousdale M. Community care of corneal ulcers. *Am J Ophthalmol.* 1992;114(5):531-538.
2. Charukamnoetkanok P, Pineda R 2nd. Controversies in management of bacterial keratitis. *Int Ophthalmol Clin.* 2005;45(4):199-210.
3. Wilhelmus K, Liesegang TJ, Osato MS, Jones DB. *Laboratory Diagnosis of Ocular Infections.* Washington, DC: American Society for Microbiology; 1994.
4. Badenoch PR, Coster DJ. Antimicrobial activity of topical anaesthetic preparations. *Br J Ophthalmol.* 1982;66(6):364-367.
5. Labetoulle M, Frau E, Offret H, Nordmann P, Naas T. Non-preserved 1% lidocaine solution has less antibacterial properties than currently available anaesthetic eye-drops. *Curr Eye Res.* 2002;25(2):91-97.
6. O'Brien TP. Bacterial keratitis. In: Foster CS, Azar DT, Dohlman CH, eds. *Smolin and Thoft's The Cornea: Scientific Foundations and Clinical Practice.* 4th ed. Philadelphia, PA: Lippincott Williams & Wilkins; 2005:235-288.
7. Waxman E, Chechelnitsky M, Mannis MJ, Schwab IR. Single culture media in infectious keratitis. *Cornea.* 1999;18(3):257-261.
8. Kaye SB, Rao PG, Smith G, et al. Simplifying collection of corneal specimens in cases of suspected bacterial keratitis. *J Clin Microbiol.* 2003;41(7):3192-3197.
9. McLeod SD, Kumar A, Cevallos V, Srinivasan M, Whitcher JP. Reliability of transport medium in the laboratory evaluation of corneal ulcers. *Am J Ophthalmol.* 2005;140(6):1027-1031.
10. Marangon FB, Miller D, Alfonso EC. Impact of prior therapy on the recovery and frequency of corneal pathogens. *Cornea.* 2004;23(2):158-164.
11. McLeod SD, Kolahdouz-Isfahani A, Rostamian K, Flowers CW, Lee PP, McDonnell PJ. The role of smears, cultures, and antibiotic sensitivity testing in the management of suspected infectious keratitis. *Ophthalmology.* 1996;103(1):23-28.
12. Rudolph T, Welinder-Olsson C, Lind-Brandberg L, Stenevi U. 16S rDNA PCR analysis of infectious keratitis: a case series. *Acta Ophthalmol Scand.* 2004;82(4):463-467.
13. Butler TK, Spencer NA, Chan CC, Singh Gilhotra J, McClellan K. Infective keratitis in older patients: a 4 year review, 1998-2002. *Br J Ophthalmol.* 2005;89(5):591-596.
14. Newton C, Moore MB, Kaufman HE. Corneal biopsy in chronic keratitis. *Arch Ophthalmol.* 1987;105(4):577-578.
15. Alexandrakis G, Haimovici R, Miller D, Alfonso EC. Corneal biopsy in the management of progressive microbial keratitis. *Am J Ophthalmol.* 2000;129(5):571-576.
16. Hwang DG. Lamellar flap corneal biopsy. *Ophthalmic Surg.* 1993;24(8):512-515.

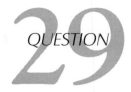

A CORNEAL INFILTRATE IS UNRESPONSIVE TO TOPICAL FLUOROQUINOLONES. COULD THIS BE ACANTHAMOEBA?

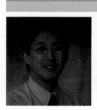

Elmer Y. Tu, MD

Acanthamoebae are free-living amoebae that form a resilient thick-walled cyst in harsh conditions. Keratitis is the most common human disease associated with *acanthamoeba* and should be considered in any patient with a corneal infiltrate that does not respond appropriately to traditional topical antibiotics because neither form is sensitive to these agents. Suspicion should be especially acute in contact lens-related (>85% to 90% of *acanthamoeba* keratitis (AK) cases in Western countries) infiltrates and/or exposure to non-sterile water as well as outdoor trauma.[1] However, fluoroquinolone resistance is not restricted to acanthamoeba, so this differential must include viral, fungal, other parasitic, and increasingly fluoroquinolone-resistant bacterial pathogens such as *Streptococcus species* and methicillin-resistant Staphylococcus aureus (MRSA).

Evaluation and Diagnosis

The clinical presentation of AK may range from diffuse epitheliitis, mild foreign body sensation with little or no stromal involvement (Figure 29-1) to the stromal ring-shaped infiltrate, radial keratoneuritis, and severe intractable pain nearly diagnostic of the infection (Figure 29-2). Disease is bilateral in up to 10% of AK and may be polymicrobial, previously identified concomitantly with viral, fungal, and bacterial pathogens.[2] Because of the specificity and long duration of therapy, definitive microbiologic diagnosis is preferred, including histologic smears of corneal scrapings (Giemsa, Wright, Diff-Quik, KOH prep,

Figure 29-1. Slit-lamp photo of a contact lens wearer with AK clinically restricted to the epithelial layer. Smears and confocal microscopy were grossly positive for the organism.

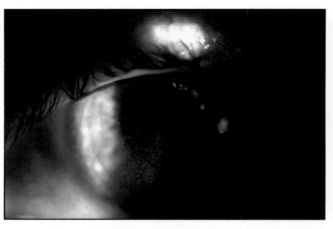

Figure 29-2. Slit-lamp photo of advanced *acanthamoeba* keratitis showing a classic immune ring infiltrate with central haze and minimal necrosis nearly pathognomonic for AK.

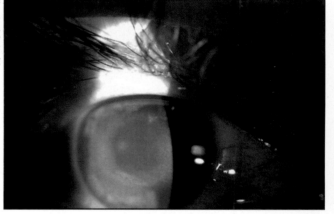

Calcafluor White, and others) or culture (non-nutrient agar with *Enterobacter* overlay). Of these methods, sensitivity and specificity is highest for histologic methods, while cultures are positive in only 0% to 50% of clinical cases of AK.[3] Corneal biopsy or polymerase chain reaction (PCR) may also be considered.

Confocal microscopy has been extensively used in the diagnosis of AK. Two units are currently available, the Confoscan 4 (Nidek Technologies, Padova, Italy) and the HRT Rostock Corneal Module (Heidelberg Engineering, Heidelberg, Germany), both of which offer *en face* serial sections of the cornea with high magnification and resolution, allowing in vivo imaging at a cellular level. Cysts are characteristically bright reflective circular opacities, sometimes with internal structures visible (Figure 29-3). In centers familiar with its use, sensitivity and specificity of confocal microscopy in the diagnosis may both exceed 90%.[3] Other imaging modalities have limited utility in AK.

Management

In the United States, no commercially available topical medications are effective for AK. We strongly recommend mechanical debridement of any clinically involved epithelium to debulk the infectious load and obtain tissue samples. Rarely, this alone may be curative in

Figure 29-3. Confocal microscopy showing multiple bright centered cysts in the anterior stroma (upper and right portions of the scan). Note that the appearance varies significantly with lighting and position.

epitheliitis, but we only use this as an adjunct to specific medical therapy. Primary topical therapy for AK is either chlorhexidine gluconate 0.02% (CHG) or polyhexamethylene biguanide 0.02% (PHMB) (Bacquacil), available only from ophthalmic compounding pharmacies. We maintain hourly dosing for the first 3 to 7 days with a gradual taper over the first month to 4 times a day, continued for several months with a more gradual taper. However, the management is highly dependent on response to these medications with some patients treated for as little as a few weeks and others, usually those with deeper stromal involvement, requiring frequent dosing for an extended period of time. Because these agents have similar mechanisms of action, we do not commonly use them together, preferring to vary concentration and/or frequency. We prefer CHG because it is better tolerated and can be increased in concentration to 0.04% or 0.06% if needed,[4] although some AK will be more responsive to a change to PHMB.

The diamidines, propamidine isethionate 0.1% (Brolene) and hexamidine isethionate 0.1% (Desmodine), are mostly effective against the trophozoites and are prescribed hourly for the first few days with a rapid taper over the first month before surface toxicity ensues. Other previously described topical agents (eg, neomycin, clotrimazole, etc) have no role in our current treatment algorithm for routine AK.

When Should Systemic Therapy, Steroids, or Therapeutic Keratoplasty Be Considered?

Because topical therapy is usually sufficient, routine systemic therapy is unnecessary. In advanced or poorly responding cases of AK, oral itraconazole (suspension preferred for greater absorption) has been described, although our own experience has been disappointing. Intravenous pentamidine and some of the newer systemic antifungals may be more effective but have not been extensively studied. Therapeutic keratoplasty is successful in recalcitrant cases or in impending perforations but with a guarded prognosis for failure, secondary glaucoma, and recurrent infection. The role of corticosteroids, both topical and systemic, is controversial with no clear evidence of detrimental effect on final outcome. Practically, we attempt to rapidly discontinue, or reduce to the lowest effective level, topical and systemic corticosteroids in patients presenting with AK. Because most extracorneal manifestations of AK are thought to be inflammatory, we will add or continue corticosteroids in cases of intractable limbitis, scleritis, and/or uveitis unresponsive to anti-acanthamoebal therapy.

How Should the Clinical Response Be Assessed and Duration of Treatment Determined?

The assessment of clinical response can be challenging in AK. The presence of epithelial infestation and radial keratoneuritis is easy to assess and usually resolves rapidly, although radial keratoneuritis may uncommonly scar exuberantly. Stromal disease is more difficult to evaluate because the borders of the keratitis are diffuse and inflammation does not always correlate with infectious activity. While some cases of post-infectious sterile corneal inflammation have been described, persistent keratitis, unlike the extracorneal manifestations, should be considered infectious unless proven otherwise. When corticosteroids are used, a constant level should be maintained to permit interval assessments of inflammatory activity as an indirect indicator of disease activity. It should be noted that viable amoeba have been recovered months to years after initial symptoms, but usually with continuing treatment. By convention, a period of 3 months of quiescence off of all medications should be observed before cure is assumed, but recurrences may rarely occur after this period.

References

1. Radford CF, Minassian DC, Dart JKG. Acanthamoeba keratitis in England and Wales: incidence, outcome, and risk factors. *Br J Ophthalmol.* May 2002;86(5):536-542.
2. Tu EY, Joslin CE, Sugar J, Shoff ME, Booton GC. Prognostic factors affecting visual outcome in Acanthamoeba keratitis. *Ophthalmology.* 2008;115(11):1998-2003.
3. Tu EY, Joslin CE, Sugar J, Booton GC, Shoff ME, Fuerst PA. The relative value of confocal microscopy and superficial corneal scrapings in the diagnosis of Acanthamoeba keratitis. *Cornea.* 2008;27(7):764-772.
4. Mathers W. Use of higher medication concentrations in the treatment of acanthamoeba keratitis. *Arch Ophthalmol.* 2006;124(6):923.

A Corneal Infiltrate of a Farmer Hit by a Tree Branch Is Not Clearing on Topical Fluoroquinolone Drops. What Should I Do Next?

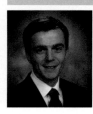

Erik Letko, MD

This patient is at risk for infectious keratitis—bacterial, fungal, or both. Corneal injury with an organic matter, such as a tree branch in this case, increases the suspicion of fungal infection. One should keep this possibility in mind at the initial visit and during the follow-up period, particularly if the patient does not respond to empiric topical antibiotics.

Epidemiology

The most common risk factors for fungal keratitis include corneal trauma with organic matter, eye conditions including prior penetrating keratoplasty, ocular surface pathology, contact lens wear, use of corticosteroids, and systemic conditions such as diabetes mellitus, compromised immune system, chronic illness, or hospitalization. According to one report, the rate of contact lens-related keratitis doubled in recent years.[1] It is noteworthy that the incidence of fungal keratitis is higher in places with a warm and humid climate. A detailed medical and ocular history and examination play a critical role in assessing the degree of suspicion of fungal keratitis. Fungal keratitis varies depending on geographic region between 6% and 20% of all infectious keratitis cases in the United States.[2] Aspergillus (Figure 30-1), Candida, and Fusarium species are the most common pathogens.

Figure 30-1. Aspergillus keratitis. Note the irregular surface of the lesion.

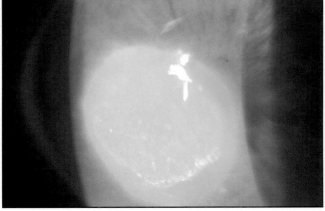

Signs and Symptoms

The symptoms of fungal keratitis typically do not present as acutely as those of bacterial keratitis. Clinical signs can vary widely, but certain slit-lamp findings such as corneal lesions with feathery margins, satellite or branching lesions, irregular surface, or intact epithelium are suspicious of fungal keratitis. One should keep in mind, however, that all of these findings could be present with bacterial keratitis. Therefore, the presence of any or all of these signs raises the likelihood of fungal keratitis, but does not confirm it. For these reasons, the diagnosis of fungal keratitis represents a challenge and is heavily dependent on laboratory methods.

Diagnosis

Harvesting a good specimen for stains and cultures plays a critical role in prompt diagnosis and treatment. The specimen should be obtained using a metal instrument, such as a spatula or surgical blade. The surgical blade might be preferable in cases where deeper scraping is needed. The specimen should contain a good sample of corneal epithelium and stroma from the area of the lesion. Removal of the involved epithelium and stroma plays not only a diagnostic, but also a therapeutic, role. In addition to gram stain used by most microbiology laboratories routinely, special stains such as Giemsa and/or calcofluor may increase the chance of identifying fungus. The culture media should include sheep blood agar, Sabouraud agar, chocolate agar, and thioglycollate broth. Although not routinely used, brain-heart infusion broth could be requested to increase the diagnostic yield, particularly when routine cultures were negative and degree of suspicion remains high.

In cases where stains and cultures of specimens scraped from the cornea were negative, corneal biopsy is indicated. If available, confocal microscopy can also be helpful. The biopsy could be performed with a 2- or 3-mm dermatologic trephine, lamellar keratectomy, or by passing a needle or suture through the involved stroma. The biopsy specimen should involve the infiltrated as well as normal tissue. It is important to keep in mind that fungi can penetrate intact Descemet's membrane and that, in the presence of hypopyon or posterior corneal plaque, anterior chamber tap may help address the question of whether fungus invaded intraocularly. These diagnostic tools are important not only in establishing the diagnosis, but also in guiding the treatment.

Treatment

Difficulties with diagnosis, lack of commercially available topical antifungal agents, and poor penetration of these agents to deeper layers of the cornea, particularly if the epithelium is intact, represent challenges when treating fungal keratitis. The most common antifungal topical agents include polyenes (natamycin and amphotericin B) and azoles (eg, ketoconazole and voriconazole). Additionally, antiseptics such as polyhexamethylene biguanide, povidone-iodine, and chlorhexidine showed some effect against fungal pathogens, but the literature data are limited.

Pimaricin (Natamycin), the only commercially available antifungal eye drops in the United States, is typically used as a first-line agent once diagnosis of fungal keratitis is established. Amphotericin B (for Candida keratitis) and an azole (for Aspergillus keratitis) can be added as a second agent, particularly in cases where response to natamycin is not satisfactory. Intraocular antifungal agents can be used at the time of anterior chamber or vitreous tap in cases where suspicion of endophthalmitis exists. The use of systemic antifungal agents has to be judicial because their therapeutic effect on fungal keratitis or endophthalmitis is limited due to poor penetration and systemic side effect profile. Systemic use of voriconazole showed some promise in a recent study.[3] The length of treatment for fungal keratitis varies widely depending on response. The minimum length of treatment is typically 1 month, but it is not unusual to use antifungal agents for several months. Repeat cultures or corneal biopsy might help determine when it is safe to cease the therapy. In cases that do not respond to antifungal agents, therapeutic keratoplasty might be needed.

Fungal keratitis represents diagnostic and therapeutic challenges. A thorough history, examination, and multiple diagnostic tests, often repeated, are required to establish the diagnosis and monitor treatment.

References

1. Jurkunas U, Behlau I, Colby K. Fungal keratitis: changing pathogens and risk factors. *Cornea.* 2009;28(6):638-643.
2. Alfonso EC, Rosa RH, Miller D. Fungal keratitis. In: Krachmer JH, Mannis MJ, Holland EJ, eds. *Cornea.* 2nd ed. Philadelphia, PA: Elsevier Mosby; 2005:1101-1114.
3. Bunya VY, Hammersmith KM, Rapuano CJ, Ayres BD, Cohen EJ. Topical and oral voriconazole in the treatment of fungal keratitis. *Am J Ophthalmol.* 2007;143(1):151-153.

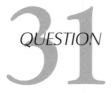

QUESTION

31

I Have a Patient With Shingles Over the Right Side of His Face and Around the Eye Treated With Oral Antivirals for 10 Days. Does This Protect Him From Eye Involvement?

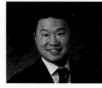

Terry Kim, MD
(co-authored with Tanya Khan, BA)

The standard treatment for herpes zoster is 7 to 10 days of oral acyclovir at a dose of 800 mg taken 5 times daily. This regimen is most effective if started within 72 hours of the onset of rash. Studies show that acyclovir administration during these first 3 days plays a preventative role by reducing viral shedding and decreasing the incidence of late ocular complications (ie, stromal keratitis, anterior uveitis) from nearly 50% to 20% to 30%.[1] Therefore, although viral spread should be static in this patient, initial treatment with oral acyclovir may not protect him from eye involvement, which can manifest shortly afterwards.

Varicella zoster virus (VZV) is one of 8 DNA herpes viruses that cause disease in humans. In its most common manifestation as childhood chickenpox, VZV characteristically causes vesicular, pruritic, disseminated lesions at varying stages of maturity. Once the primary infection resolves clinically, VZV can remain dormant in the trigeminal and dorsal root ganglia for a period of years to decades. Under appropriate conditions of stress (ie, immunosuppression, aging), the virus reactivates as a unilateral vesicular eruption within a dermatomal distribution. This presentation is known as herpes zoster, or shingles. When the first division of the trigeminal nerve (ie, ophthalmic nerve) is involved, infection can spread to the eye and result in herpes zoster ophthalmicus (HZO).[2]

How Does Eye Involvement Present and How Often Should the Patient Be Examined?

The typical presentation of HZO begins with a prodromal phase of influenza-like symptoms, including fatigue, low-grade fever, and malaise. These symptoms can be present up to 1 week before a rash appears over the forehead, followed by the rapid development of midline-observing lesions in the corresponding dermatome of the ophthalmic nerve. At this point, the virus can infect the globe via the nasociliary branch of the ophthalmic nerve. You should begin to consider eye involvement with signs suggestive of blepharoconjunctivitis as this is usually the earliest ocular finding of herpes zoster. Upon initial suspicion, plan to see the patient back within 1 week to monitor for keratitis or keratouveitis, which can develop as early as 1 to 2 days after the appearance of a rash (punctate epithelial keratitis) and as late as 1 month following the rash (deep stromal keratitis).

Differentiating Herpes Zoster From Herpes Simplex

Varicella zoster virus and the herpes simplex virus (HSV) belong to the same family of Herpesviridae. Both viruses can cause corneal inflammation and clinically present in a similar fashion, with the common symptoms being pain, photophobia, and blurred vision. The key distinction between the two lies in their appearances on slit-lamp examination. Herpes zoster virus dendrites are infiltrative and branch into medusa-like patterns with tapered ends, whereas herpes simplex virus dendrites are ulcerative and terminate into bulbs.

Treatment Options

It is important to correctly identify the causative viral agent because doing so will directly affect how you manage your patient's disease. For herpes simplex epithelial keratitis, topical antivirals (ie, trifluorothymidine 1% solution administered 9 times daily and/or vidarabine 3% ointment [available in Canada, in Europe, and in the United States under limited pharmaceutical coverage] administered 5 times daily) are the mainstays of treatment. Alternatively, oral acyclovir at a dose of 400 mg taken 5 times daily for 7 to 10 days has been reported to be as effective as topical antivirals with the added benefit of no ocular toxicity, an adverse outcome that has been previously associated with topical antiviral therapy. The prophylactic maintenance dose of 400 mg oral acyclovir taken twice daily has been used off-label to treat epithelial HSV disease, especially if the patient is prone to surface epithelial toxicity.

Oral antiviral therapy for HZO is not typically continued beyond 10 days; however, you should bear in mind that your particularly immunocompromised and elderly patients may require a longer course of treatment because the viral DNA can persist in the cornea for up to 30 days. Also consider prolonged antiviral therapy when treating serious complications, such as retinal involvement. Treat blepharoconjunctivitis palliatively with cool compresses and frequent topical lubrication. With skin involvement, consider adding topical antibiotics (ie, bacitracin, gentamicin, or moxifloxacin) to the treatment regimen.

Complications

A frequent complication of HZO to be aware of is anterior keratouveitis. Common signs of uveitis include redness, photophobia, blurred vision, and irregular pupil. HZV keratouveitis may be recurrent or chronic and can lead to iris atrophy, glaucoma, and cataract formation. Remember that HSV-related iris atrophy is usually observed near the pupillary sphincter whereas HZO-related iris atrophy is more basal, segmental, and due to iris stromal occlusive vasculitis. The recommendation for uveitis management is topical steroids (eg, prednisolone acetate 1% 4 times daily) and cycloplegic drops (homatropine 5% 3 to 4 times daily or scopolamine 0.25% 2 to 4 times daily).

Because of the associated anterior segment inflammation, these patients often develop visually significant cataracts sooner than the normal population. Often, cataract surgery is more complicated due to corneal scarring, abnormal iris/pupil, posterior synechiae, as well as postoperative inflammation. These issues should be addressed with the patient, along with appropriate surgical planning.

The most significant long-term consequence of HZO is corneal disease, which occurs in approximately 40% of all cases.[3] Such patients often complain of decreased vision, photosensitivity, and pain. As the virus penetrates the epithelium and stroma, cumulative damage weakens the cornea, resulting in delayed epithelial healing and increased susceptibility to microtrauma. With continued progression, substantial corneal scarring can result, potentially leading to corneal thinning and perforation. In this scenario, you may need to discuss the possibility of full- or partial-thickness corneal transplantation with your patient. It is important to advise the patient that corneal sensitivity will decrease immediately following surgery but may slowly and partially recover with time. These patients should also be aware that vision is very difficult to predict following keratoplasty and that several months may pass before selective suture removal takes place for visual rehabilitation. Finally, these patients should know that once suture removal is completed, glasses and/or contact lenses may still be required to improve vision following transplantation and that irregular astigmatism and/or anisometropia may limit the quality of vision. Many of these transplant patients are also placed on long-term topical corticosteroid medication to help prevent the development of neovascularization, associated lipid deposition, and graft rejection that can develop months or even years after successful surgery.

Is Vaccination Helpful?

The role of vaccination in herpes zoster prevention has been established for some time, but not much is known regarding its specific value in precluding the development of ophthalmologic sequelae. The herpes zoster vaccine contains live, attenuated varicella virus that induces protection 70% to 90% of the time. It has been shown to greatly bolster cell-mediated immunity and thereby reduce the probability of VZV reactivation. It is recommended that adults over the age of 60 years receive the vaccine. Although increasing evidence from both the Herpetic Eye Disease Study and Uchoa and colleagues shows that oral acyclovir use (400 mg twice daily) for at least 12 months substantially reduces the number of recurrences of herpes simplex ocular infection,[4,5] there is no evidence to date to support the prophylactic use of acyclovir or other antiviral medication in case of herpes zoster ophthalmicus. Similarly, to date, diet modification plays no known role in herpes zoster prevention.

References

1. Gnann JW, Whitley RJ. Herpes zoster. *N Engl J Med*. 2002;347(5):340-346.
2. Shaikh S, Ta CN. Evaluation and management of herpes zoster ophthalmicus. *Am Fam Physician*. 2002;66(9):1723-1730.
3. Arffa RC. Viral diseases. In: Arffa RC, Grayson M, eds. *Grayson's Diseases of the Cornea*. 4th ed. St. Louis, MO: Mosby; 1997:283-337.
4. Herpetic Eye Disease Study Group. Oral acyclovir for herpes simplex virus eye disease: effect on prevention of epithelial keratitis and stromal keratitis. *Arch Ophthalmol*. 2000;118(8):1030-1036.
5. Uchoa UBC, Rezende RA, Carrasco MA, Rapuano CJ, Laibson PR, Cohen EJ. Long-term acyclovir use to prevent recurrent ocular herpes simplex virus infection. *Arch Ophthalmol*. 2003;121(12):1702-1704.

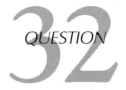

QUESTION

32

I HAVE A PATIENT WITH HERPES SIMPLEX DENDRITES. WHAT IS THE BEST PLAN TO MINIMIZE BOTH THE RECURRENCES AND POSSIBLE SCARRING?

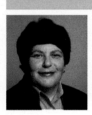

Penny Asbell, MD, FACS, MBA
(co-authored with Daniel Brocks, MD)

The large, well-organized Herpetic Eye Disease Study (HEDS) has guided our treatment of herpes simplex keratitis (Figure 32-1). It is clear from these investigations that initial treatment of herpes simplex epithelial keratitis with a topical antiviral, such as trifluridine, hastens the healing process. In addition, HEDS suggested that oral antiviral, in addition to topical antiviral, treatment did not provide any additional benefit for treating dendritic keratitis, such as increasing healing time or preventing possible additional corneal or intraocular involvement including stromal keratitis or iridocyclitis.[1,2]

The appropriate treatment to attempt to prevent recurrence requires a review of the findings of the HEDS—Acyclovir Prevention Trial. The study goal was to investigate the use of oral acyclovir 400 mg twice a day for 1 year versus placebo to assess the time to a recurrence of herpetic eye disease. The results showed that the oral acyclovir treatment reduced the rate of recurrence of herpetic eye disease by 41% in those patients who had any form of HSV infection of the eye in the past year. In addition, the rate of stromal keratitis was cut in half in those patients who specifically had stromal keratitis in the past year.[3]

Less clear data are available regarding the use of mechanical debridement of the epithelium. A Cochrane database review revealed equivocal data as to whether adding debridement to a regimen of antiviral treatment had any benefit over topical antiviral treatment alone.[4]

Overall, our routine care for patients with herpes simplex epithelial keratitis includes topical antivirals followed by a discussion with the patient regarding the usefulness of

Figure 32-1. HSV epithelial keratitis with terminal bulbs in patient 1 year status post-PRK. Without fluorescein staining (A) and after fluorescein staining (B).

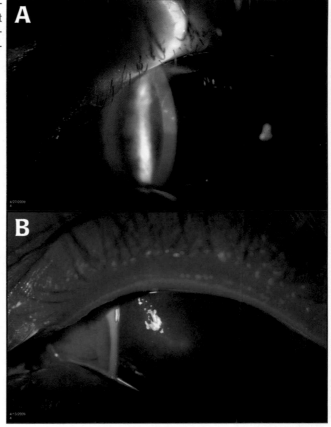

prophylaxis against recurrent disease with the use of oral antivirals. Because most episodes of dendritic keratitis resolve without loss of vision, I generally do not suggest oral antivirals to prevent recurrences. If the patient chooses to start antivirals, it need not be started until the current episode has resolved, as there has been no benefit found in using both topical and oral antivirals in the treatment of a current episode of herpetic epithelial keratitis.

Management of Disciform Keratitis and Stromal Scarring

Disciform keratitis and stromal scarring (Figures 32-2 and 32-3) is also handled using information predominantly obtained from HEDS.[5] The treatment of stromal keratitis was clearly shown to benefit from the addition of topical prednisolone phosphate 1% eye drops tapered over 10 weeks along with topical trifluridine. These patients, when compared to those who received placebo (artificial tears), had faster resolution of their stromal inflammation and showed no significant increase in recurrence rates. It is of vital importance to note that none of these patients had any active HSV epithelial keratitis. In addition, the use of oral acyclovir with the topical steroid/trifluridine regimen was reviewed, and no significant advantage was found with adding the oral medication. Using this information, we routinely treat these patients with the topical trifluridine/steroid combination. We generally

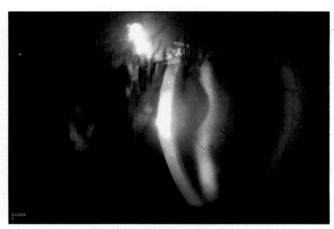

Figure 32-2. Active HSV stromal keratitis with keratitic precipitates.

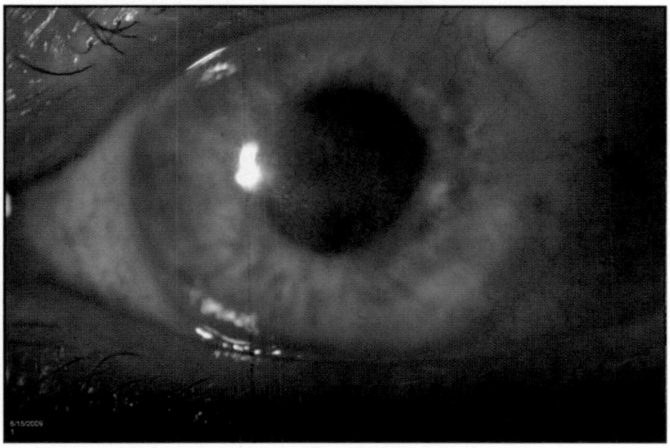

Figure 32-3. Limbal neovascularization status post-HSV keratitis with residual central stromal scar. Some have advocated the use of bevacizumab topical eye drop treatment in these patients to treat neovascularization.

recommend topical prednisolone acetate 1% and trifluridine used about 4 times a day each and then tapered at the same rate, slowly to prevent reactivation. The drops should be tapered together—for example, when prednisolone is decreased to 3 times a day, trifluridine should be decreased to 3 times a day as well. In addition, some patients may need a chronic dose of steroid in a very low dose, such as used only 2 or 3 times per week. Ideally, the trifluridine should be continued until the patient is off of prednisolone drops. It is important to follow these patients for evidence of medication toxicity from the use of trifluridine and to taper or stop this drop as the healing process advances. The later addition of oral acyclovir when the acute process has resolved should be discussed with the patient and may be started to decrease the risk of recurrences. Because stromal keratitis can cause corneal scarring and permanent loss of vision, prevention of recurrences is important and the use of oral antivirals is always discussed. Risks of oral antivirals are generally minimal and include diarrhea, nausea, and headache, but they can be more severe (ie, hepatitis and renal impairment). Given the likelihood of long-term use, I suggest ruling out liver disease and impaired renal function prior to use and regular evaluation of serum liver and kidney function tests while on the medication. Avoidance is recommended if pregnancy for the patient or partner is planned, and avoidance if nursing is recommended. It should be noted that the effect of acyclovir to reduce recurrences only works while taking acyclovir, and if discontinued, the risk of recurrence is no longer reduced.

New and Alternative Treatments

Research into alternative, more effective treatments is ongoing. Gancyclovir used topically, which is approved in Europe, is currently being studied in the United States. Research into the use of helicase/primase inhibitors or Toll-like receptor agonists (ie, imiquimod, resiquimod) is ongoing. Of particular interest is the quest for an intervention that can prevent or eradicate HSV infection rather than simply suppress recurrent episodes, which occur due to the ability of the virus to remain latent within the body. Within this category, research on therapeutic vaccines and preventative vaccines has grown. Vaccines made from heat-killed HSV-1 and HSV-2, an inactivated subunit vaccine containing mixed HSV-2 subunits and a recombinant glycoprotein vaccine, have so far shown no statistically significant results in terms of prevention of recurrences or decreasing duration of recurrences. Some promising results have been found in recent studies of a live attenuated vaccine in clinical trials in preventing virus reactivation, but continued research is needed.[6]

There are not sufficient data to come to a conclusion regarding whether diet modification plays a role in the treatment or prevention of HSV keratitis. Several animal models have shown that poor diet (malnourishment) may play an important role in the ability to heal after an HSV infection.[7] Other environmental factors were evaluated in the HEDS recurrence factor study. Specifically, patients with HSV ocular disease in the previous year were followed with a weekly questionnaire reviewing several study factors and reported whether ocular disease recurred. The study showed there were no clear external factors (including psychological stress, systemic infection, UV exposure, contact lens wear, menstrual cycle, eye injury) that were associated with HSV ocular recurrence.[8] Interestingly, a recent case report described an episode of herpes epithelial keratitis and iritis 5 days following corneal cross-linking with riboflavin and ultraviolet A for keratoconus.[9] Recurrent HSV has been reported post-refractive laser treatment (LASIK, PRK), and oral antivirals have been shown to be effective in preventing post-laser exposure HSV recurrences in an animal model.[10]

Long-Term Use of Antivirals

Although the HEDS—Acyclovir Prevention Trial showed that the use of oral acyclovir for 1 year decreased recurrence rates in those patients who had previous HSV ocular disease in the preceding year, it did not answer the question of how long patients should remain on oral antivirals. A 2003 retrospective study at Wills Eye Hospital seemed to indicate that the use of oral acyclovir beyond 12 months continued to have efficacy in preventing ocular herpes recurrences.[11] The lack of information from a large population studied past 12 months of use must be reviewed with the patient, along with the risks, although fairly low for most patients, of long-term acyclovir systemic treatment. Overall, there does seem to be a role for long-term use of oral acyclovir, particularly making sense in patients with a history of recurrent disease off acyclovir that has affected vision.

References

1. The Herpetic Eye Disease Study Group. A controlled trial of oral acyclovir for the prevention of stromal keratitis or iritis in patients with herpes simplex virus epithelial keratitis. *Arch Ophthalmol.* 1997;115(6):703-712.
2. Sudesh S, Laibson PR. The impact of the Herpetic Eye Disease Studies on the management of herpes simplex virus ocular infections. *Curr Opin Ophthalmol.* 1999;10(4):230-233.
3. Barron BA, Gee L, Hauck WW, et al. Herpetic Eye Disease Study. A controlled trial of oral acyclovir for herpes simplex stromal keratitis. *Ophthalmology.* 1994;101(12):1871-1882.
4. Wilhelmus KR. Interventions for herpes simplex virus epithelial keratitis. *Cochrane Database Syst Rev.* 2003;(3):CD002898.
5. Wilhelmus KR, Gee L, Hauck WW, et al. Herpetic Eye Disease Study. A controlled trial of topical corticosteroids for herpes simplex stromal keratitis. *Ophthalmology.* 1994;101(12):1883-1895.
6. Wilson SS, Fakioglu E, Harold BC. Novel approaches in fighting herpes simplex virus infections. *Expert Rev Anti Infect Ther.* 2009;7(5):559-568.
7. Benencia F, Gamba G, Benedetti R, Courreges MC, Cavalieri H, Massouh EJ. Effect of undernourishment on Herpes Simplex Virus Type 1 ocular infection in the Wistar rat model. *Int J Exp Pathol.* 2002;83(2):57-66.
8. Herpetic Eye Disease Study Group. Psychological Stress and other potential triggers for recurrences of herpes simplex virus eye infections. *Arch Ophthalmol.* 2000;118(12):1617-1625.
9. Kymionis GD, Portaliou DM, Bouzoukis DI, et al. Herpetic keratitis with iritis after corneal crosslinking with riboflavin and ultraviolet A for keratoconus. *J Cataract Refract Surg.* 2007;33(11):1982-1984.
10. Asbell PA. Valacyclovir for the prevention of recurrent herpes simplex virus eye disease after excimer laser photokeratectomy. *Trans Am Ophthalmol Soc.* 2000;98:285-303.
11. Uchoa UB, Rezende RA, Carrasco MA, Rapuano CJ, Laibson PR, Cohen EJ. Long-term acyclovir use to prevent recurrent ocular herpes simplex virus infection. *Arch Ophthalmol.* 2003;121(12):1702-1704.

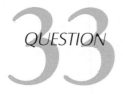
AFTER RECENTLY TREATED BACTERIAL KERATITIS, A DIABETIC PATIENT CONTINUES TO HAVE PERSISTENT STROMAL ULCER DESPITE BANDAGE CONTACT LENS AND TOPICAL ANTIBIOTICS. WHAT ARE THE OPTIONS?

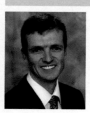

Carlindo Da Reitz Pereira, MD

A non-healing persistent epithelial defect or sterile ulcer often tends to have a prolonged course. Besides causing frustration to both the clinician and the patient, it can have devastating visual and ocular outcomes if it is not treated promptly and effectively.

Differential Diagnosis

A careful history can often give clues to an underlying mechanism responsible for the persistent epithelial defect or sterile ulcer. Identifying the potential underlying cause is important as it allows for a more definitive and effective treatment, which can prevent blinding consequences. Table 33-1 summarizes reported causes that are important not to miss.

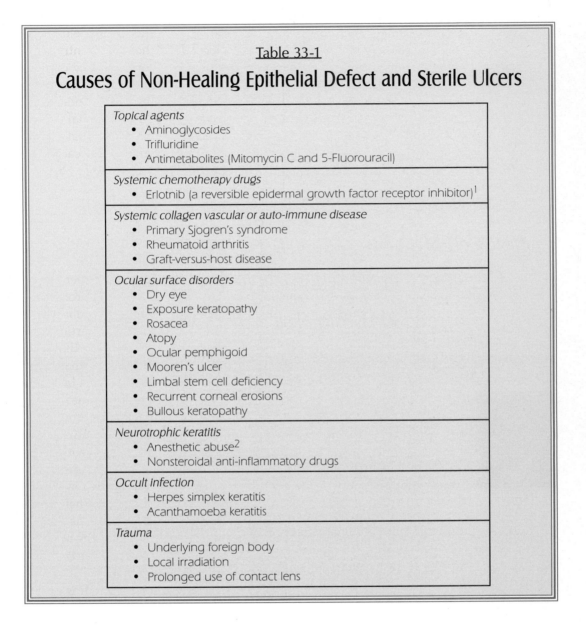

Table 33-1

Causes of Non-Healing Epithelial Defect and Sterile Ulcers

Topical agents
- Aminoglycosides
- Trifluridine
- Antimetabolites (Mitomycin C and 5-Fluorouracil)

Systemic chemotherapy drugs
- Erlotnib (a reversible epidermal growth factor receptor inhibitor)[1]

Systemic collagen vascular or auto-immune disease
- Primary Sjogren's syndrome
- Rheumatoid arthritis
- Graft-versus-host disease

Ocular surface disorders
- Dry eye
- Exposure keratopathy
- Rosacea
- Atopy
- Ocular pemphigoid
- Mooren's ulcer
- Limbal stem cell deficiency
- Recurrent corneal erosions
- Bullous keratopathy

Neurotrophic keratitis
- Anesthetic abuse[2]
- Nonsteroidal anti-inflammatory drugs

Occult infection
- Herpes simplex keratitis
- Acanthamoeba keratitis

Trauma
- Underlying foreign body
- Local irradiation
- Prolonged use of contact lens

Examination

Evaluate externally for proptosis, lagophthalmos, floppy eyelid syndrome, and decreased blink rate, which may cause exposure. Be sure not to miss something as simple as a small foreign body that may be buried in the base of the sterile ulcer or lodged under the eyelids. Conjunctival injection that tends to predominantly involve the inferior conjunctiva and fornix is suggestive of medicamentosa. Evaluate the corneal epithelium for any signs of basement-membrane dystrophy, which may cause recurrent erosions. The location and shape of the epithelial defect can also offer clues to the underlying process. Peripheral epithelial defects or ulcers are more likely related to immune-related causes.

A superior oval ulcer is suggestive of vernal keratoconjunctivitis-induced Shield ulcer. An oval or scaphoid-shaped epithelial defect or ulcer located in the inferocentral cornea is classic for neurotrophic keratitis (Figure 33-1). This can be confirmed by corneal sensation, ideally using an esthesiometer or thin cotton fibers to quantify the sensation. Performing a Schirmer's test with anesthesia is also important to identify an underlying tear production deficiency. Look for any elevated tissue adjacent to the epithelial defect, such as a raised pterygium or bleb that could suggest the development of a corneal dellen. Be sure to document and follow the thickness of the underlying stromal bed at each visit to not miss stromal melting or an impending perforation.

Treatment

MEDICAL MANAGEMENT

I would obtain a corneal culture if there is any infiltrate present or if the patient is on a topical steroid that could mask an infectious process. Treatment is aimed at promoting surface healing and preventing progression of stromal melt. Stop or taper topical medications that are toxic to the epithelium, such as frequent fortified antibiotics, particularly aminoglycosides. Preservatives in eye drops are some of the biggest offenders that lead to irritation of the epithelium, causing punctate epithelial erosions. If the combination of drops being used is more than 4 to 5 times per day, the preservatives alone can be toxic. Remove offending topical agents that delay surface healing, such as topical nonsteroidal anti-inflammatory drugs, especially when used in combination with topical steroids.[3]

Apply lubricants frequently, using non-preserved artificial tears and lubricating ointment. Adding systemic omega-3 fatty acids such as flaxseed oil and fish oil with their anti-inflammatory properties may also be beneficial by decreasing pro-inflammatory cytokines and improving the quality of the tear film. For sterile ulcers, adding systemic doxycycline with its anticollagenase properties reduces the rate of corneal melts. For poorly responding epithelial defects, one can consider using autologous serum as topical eye drops, which has shown promise in decreasing healing time by suppressing apoptosis in conjunctival and corneal epithelium. Application of a bandage contact lens can also aid the healing of persistent or recurrent erosions (Figure 33-2).

If the patient has a history of prior herpetic eye disease, or for non-responding cases, I would consider adding systemic acyclovir, as herpetic keratitis may present as a non-healing epithelial defect. A topical cycloplegic agent can be used if there is any ocular pain, or a significant anterior chamber reaction.

Also consider systemic evaluation and lab workup for underlying immune disorders, as the presence of an underlying disease can be the major contributing factor.[4]

SURGICAL MANAGEMENT

I find sequential punctal occlusion, initially using non-surgical punctal plugs, helpful to treat underlying dry eye. For cases associated with severe dry eye, I perform punctal cautery, which can preclude some patients from needing a tarsorrhaphy. For sterile ulcers that are severe or that respond poorly to medical treatment, perform a lateral or central tarsorrhaphy to be left in for a few weeks. The tarsorrhaphy can later be partially opened,

Figure 33-1. Sterile ulcer in a patient with underlying severe dry eye and neurotrophic keratitis following penetrating keratoplasty, who had previously undergone lateral tarsorrhaphy.

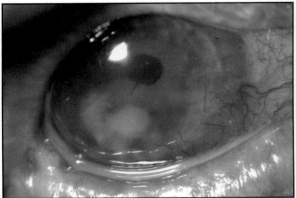

Figure 33-2. Longstanding, recurrent central corneal ulceration in a diabetic patient requiring bandage contact lens to prevent epithelial breakdown. At time of photo, epithelium is intact but anterior stroma is hazy and irregular.

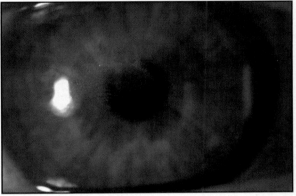

but premature opening can cause a recurrent melt. For patients who refuse a tarsorrhaphy, a Botox injection to the superior levator muscle can be used for temporary ptosis of the upper lid. An alternative to a total tarsorrhaphy is to combine a small temporal tarsorrhaphy with placement of an amniotic membrane over the defect. The amniotic membrane is cut to size and placed stromal side down on the corneal defect and secured using either fibrin glue or suturing it to the edges of the ulcer. If the ulcer has greater than 50% stromal melt, multiple layers of the amniotic membrane can be used to fill the defect, leaving the bottom layers unsutured, and suturing the very top layer to the edge of the stromal defect with 10-0 nylon. Once the defect is covered and the top layer is secured, an overlay amniotic membrane is then used basement membrane side down to cover the entire cornea, and sutured to the perilimbal conjunctiva.

For eyes with poor visual potential or in situations where the underlying condition such as exposure cannot be controlled, a conjunctival flap can be an excellent option for either short-term or long-term treatment. However, with flaps that cover the pupil area, the visual results will be limited at best.

When stromal melts progress, cyanoacrylate glue can be applied after removing loose surrounding epithelium and carefully cleaning and drying the stromal bed. Apply thin layers of glue and let it dry until the desired area is covered, then place a bandage contact lens for comfort. If these measures are not successful, the corneal melt can progress to a perforation. This will require an emergency surgery to repair the perforation with a lamellar or full-thickness tectonic graft.

References

1. Johnson KS, Levin F, Chu DS. Persistent corneal epithelial defect associated with erlotinib treatment. *Cornea.* 2009;28(6):706-707.
2. Burns RP. Toxic effects of local anesthetics. *JAMA.* 1978;240(4):347.
3. Hersch PS, Rice BA, Baer JC, et al. Topical nonsteroidal agents and corneal wound healing. *Arch Ophthalmol.* 1990;108(4):577-583.
4. Petroutsos G, Paschides CA, Kitsos G, Skopouli FN, Psilas K. Sterile corneal ulcers in dry eye. Incidence and factors of occurrence. *J Fr Ophtalmol.* 1992;15(2):103-105.

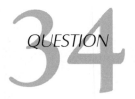

A PATIENT WITH A HISTORY OF RECURRENT HSV KERATITIS CONTINUES TO HAVE DENSE PUNCTATE KERATOPATHY AND VISUAL ACUITY OF 20/100 DESPITE HOURLY LUBRICATION WITH PRESERVATIVE-FREE ARTIFICIAL TEARS. WHAT ELSE COULD BE DONE?

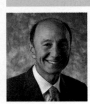

Michael W. Belin, MD

Persistent keratopathy after an episode of stromal HSV keratitis is a fairly common scenario. I think the most frequently overlooked diagnostic test is an accurate assessment of the corneal sensation. Typically, patients have a battery of screening exams before they see the physician. This necessitates the use of anesthetic drops and complicates the assessment of corneal sensation. The importance here is to separate those patients with normal sensation, decreased sensation, and no sensation (completely anesthetic cornea). While a more graded quantitative assessment can be performed with devices such as an esthesiometer (eg, Cochet-Bonnet), adequate corneal assessment can be performed using some wisps from the end of a cotton/Dacron applicator.

Examination

If the involved cornea has normal sensation (equal to the uninvolved eye), then one would be hard pressed to attribute the persistent punctate keratopathy completely to the resolved HSV, and one should look for other contributing factors. Dry eyes (often asymmetric), lid disease, and topical and/or systemic medications may cause a punctate keratitis and are not uncommon in a post-menopausal female.

The greater the number of recurrences of HSV, the greater the loss in corneal sensation. With multiple recurrences, instead of reduced sensation, patients may have no corneal sensation at all. If the patient's cornea is completely devoid of sensation, then, in my experience, nothing you do short of an aggressive tarsorrhaphy or conjunctival flap will completely resolve the problem. In these cases, mild to moderate punctate keratitis with 20/100 vision may be a reasonable and acceptable endpoint, and treatment (as discussed below) should be directed at preventing further complications. Patients should be spared unnecessary treatments when there is little potential benefit.

The following discussion is directed at the more common scenario of mild to moderate persistent punctate keratopathy associated with a mild to moderate decrease in corneal sensation following recurrent HSV keratitis. The first thing is to make sure you are treating what you think you are treating. In a patient with recurrent HSV, you must ensure that your clinical findings do not represent active disease. Because this patient has a known history of HSV recurrence, I would make sure the patient is on chronic suppressive therapy, including systemic antivirals (obviously avoid topical antivirals due to their toxicity) and a topical steroid if the patient was steroid-dependent in the past. While chronic steroids are often contraindicated in chronic surface disease, steroid-dependent HSV patients are different, and the lowest amount of steroid necessary to control inflammation should be maintained. Next, examine the other eye. Rule out other conditions that can cause epithelial keratitis such as dry eye, blepharitis, meibomitis, thyroid disease, other topical medications, and systemic medications associated with ocular surface drying. Asymmetric presentation of epithelial disease is not uncommon. In this case, however, the central location (versus the more typical inferior location) makes typical dry eye and/or exposure less likely.

Treatment

One of the important dictums in patients with neurotrophic keratitis is *"Le mieux est l'ennemi du bien"* (as quoted by Voltaire,[1] often translated as "Better is the enemy of Good"). Patient and physician expectations need to be realistic. You rarely "cure" the disease. The goal of treatment should be to maximize vision, minimize symptoms, and prevent complications without making the patient a slave to the disease. One of the most important diagnostic "tests" is to make sure that the reduction in visual acuity is attributable to the disease you are trying to treat. Mild surface disruption, such as seen with punctate keratitis, can severely affect visual performance. Patients should notice a significant improvement in visual acuity with a diagnostic rigid lens fit. If the vision does not improve significantly, alternate reasons for a reduction in vision should be evaluated.

The initial assessment should include the standard tests for dry eyes, including Schirmer's tear measurements; Lissamine green staining of the cornea and conjunctiva; and examination of the lid margins and lid function, meibomian glands, and punctae. Initial treatments typically include frequent use of non-preserved artificial tears. Additional modalities consist of thicker tear gels or Lacriserts. Patients with mild to moderate neurotrophic disease often tolerate the Lacrisert insert well. Low-dose systemic doxycycline may be added. As noted above, low-dose topical steroids can help at times. Alternately, topical 1% methylprogesterone can be used as this avoids some of the potential collagenolytic activity, but it has to be specially formulated. Patients with neurotrophic disease have mixed responses to topical 0.05% cyclosporine (Restasis), but this medication is well-tolerated and should be given an adequate trial. In my experience, topical nonsteroidals are not helpful, and the potential for corneal melts with NSAIDs should be considered.

When possible, offending systemic medications that may aggravate a dry eye (eg, antihistamines) should be eliminated or changed, and patients, when applicable, should be instructed to cease smoking. Patients should also be instructed to increase the use of tears during periods of reading and/or computer use as a reduction in the normal blink rate is typically seen in these circumstances. Other more aggressive treatments include punctal plugs, pressure patching, and tarsorrhaphy. While I am not a big user of plugs in my "normal" dry eye population, they do play a role in patients with exposure or neuro-trophic disease. Partial tarsorrhaphy is a very effective procedure and will often result in rapid resolution in spite of other earlier treatments. Patients, however, particularly those with good visual acuity in the other eye, often find the procedure cosmetically unaccept-able. Bandage contact lenses are a mixed blessing. They can often result in an improve-ment in visual acuity, but their risk is increased by the fact that minor irritations often initially go unnoticed by the patient due to the anesthetic cornea.

Other treatment modalities such as autologous serum drops, conjunctival flap, or amniotic membrane grafts are more commonly reserved for chronic non-healing epithe-lial defects and are rarely justified in patients with superficial punctate keratitis. While a well-performed thin Gunderson flap can allow reasonable visual acuity, one must ensure that the "treatment" is not worse than the disease.

Reference

1. Voltaire. *La Begueule, Conte Moral (1772)*. Whitefish, MT: Kessinger Publishing; 2009.

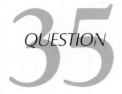
A Patient With Red, Irritated Eyes, Tearing, and Photophobia That Started Yesterday Has Mild Conjunctival Injection and 2+ Follicles of the Palpebral Conjunctiva. When the Patient Awoke, His Eyelids Were Stuck Closed. Is This Acute Conjunctivitis?

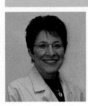

Marian Macsai, MD

The exam showed conjunctival injection, inflammation, and exudate (Figure 35-1). Conjunctivitis, or inflammation of the conjunctiva, is characterized by injection, dilated vessels, exudate, and often chemosis. In patients with acute conjunctivitis (less than 3 weeks), the history, age, duration of symptoms, clinical exam, type of exudate, and conjunctival scrapings help determine the etiology.

Acute Papillary Conjunctivitis

Conjunctival papillae, a nonspecific sign of inflammation, are caused by edema and polymorphonuclear cell infiltration.[1] The hypertrophic projections of epithelium contain a central fibrovascular core on the palpebral conjunctiva. In adult patients with acute papillary conjunctivitis and mucopurulent discharge, infection by *Staphylococcus aureus*, *Haemophilus influenzae*, and streptococci are common. Methicillin-resistant *Staphylococcus aureus* (MRSA) conjunctivitis is increasing among the nursing home population and

Figure 35-1. Acute conjunctivitis with purulent discharge on the lashes and diffuse conjunctival injection and edema.

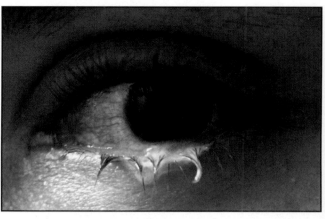

community-acquired infections.[2] *H. influenzae* conjunctivitis occurs in adults chronically colonized with the bacteria, such as smokers or patients with chronic pulmonary disease.[1] *H. influenzae* biotype III (previously called *H. aegyptuis*) presents with conjunctival hemorrhages, peripheral keratitis, and stromal infiltrates (Figure 35-2). In contrast, *S. pneumoniae* presents with inflammatory tarsal membranes and conjunctival hemorrhages. Bacterial conjunctivitis is frequently bilateral; therefore, nasolacrimal duct obstruction, dacryocystitis, or canaliculitis should be considered in an adult with a unilateral presentation. Underlying risk factors such as dry eye, exposure due to lid abnormalities, untreated blepharitis, vitamin A deficiency, or immunosuppression require evaluation and management after resolution of the initial episode.

In healthy adults, mild bacterial conjunctivitis may be self-limited, but using topical antibacterial drops is associated with earlier remission occurring in 2 to 5 days in more than 60% of patients compared with placebo.[3] My initial antibiotic choice is usually empirical, and I use polymyxin/trimethoprim drops 4 times a day for 1 week. Available as a generic, this antibiotic provides broad-spectrum coverage at a low cost to the patient, which increases compliance. Patients are instructed to follow-up in 3 to 4 days if they note no improvement. In patients who are debilitated, immunocompromised, unresponsive to initial treatment, or have severe cases of purulent conjunctivitis, I perform gram-stained smears and cultures of their conjunctiva.

In cases of acute papillary conjunctivitis with hyperpurulent discharge, Neisseria gonorrheae or N. meningitides must be suspected.[4] Patients present with massive purulent exudation, severe chemosis, and a rapidly progressive course, often less than 24 hours. If left untreated, there may be progression to corneal ulceration, perforation, and systemic meningococcal dissemination. When gonococcal infection is a possibility, gram stain and culture with chocolate agar media in a 4% to 8% CO_2 environment are done, and systemic therapy with daily follow-up is initiated. Frequent saline lavage can provide comfort, decrease inflammation, and prevent corneal melting. Patients without corneal ulceration are treated with 1 g of ceftriaxone given intramuscularly, whereas patients with corneal involvement receive intravenous ceftriaxone (1 g every 12 hours for 3 days) and a topical antibiotic ointment. Patients and sexual contacts are informed about the possibility of concomitant chlamydial disease. Additionally, sexual abuse is considered in children with this presentation.

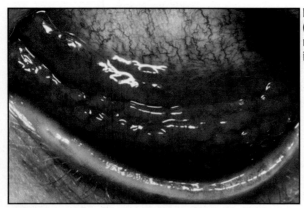

Figure 35-2. *H. influenzae* biotype III (*H. aegyptuis*) with conjunctival hemorrhages, peripheral keratitis, and stromal infiltrates.

In the pediatric population, the differential diagnosis for acute papillary conjunctivitis includes *Staphylococcus aureus, Haemophilus influenzae, S. pneumoniae*, anaerobic bacteria (*Peptostreptococcus* sp. and *Peptococcus* sp.), and *Moraxella* species.[1] *H. influenzae* can occur in association with otitis media or preseptal cellulitis, which may predispose children to a fulminant meningitis. Of note, vaccination against Hib has significantly reduced the incidence of *H. influenzae* conjunctivitis.

Acute Follicular Conjunctivitis

Acute follicular conjunctivitis may result from viral infections or early chlamydial inclusion conjunctivitis.[1] Follicles are aggregates of lymphocytes surrounded by mast cells and plasma in the superficial conjunctival stroma (Figure 35-3). Often, nonspecific concomitant papillae are present. Chlamydial infection from serotypes D-K is suspected in sexually active patients with unilateral acute conjunctivitis, scant discharge, and pre-auricular lymphadenopathy. Typically, follicles become more prominent in the second or third week of presentation. Epithelial infiltrates and micropannus involving the superior cornea may also be noted. In adult chlamydial inclusion conjunctivitis, we prescribe one oral dose of azithromycin 1000 mg or doxycycline 100 mg twice daily for 7 days.[2] Co-infection with gonorrhea and syphilis must be investigated, and all sexual partners must be treated.

A variety of viruses cause acute follicular conjunctivitis, including herpes simplex virus (HSV), Paramyxoviridae, measles, mumps, and Newcastle disease with adenovirus being the most common.[1] Adenovirus presents as follicular conjunctivitis, epidemic keratoconjunctivitis (EKC), or pharyngeal conjunctival fever (PCF). Patients with EKC typically present with follicular conjunctivitis and pre-auricular lymphadenopathy, corneal sub-epithelial infiltrates by day 10 to 14, and blurred vision or photophobia. The highly contagious nature of this disease requires patient education to avoid transmission and possible quarantine. While there is no effective treatment for EKC, the use of artificial tears, topical antihistamines, or cold compresses may provide symptomatic relief.[2] If a conjunctival membrane forms, debridement can be performed for patient comfort. Spontaneous resolution without topical steroids will occur, and patient reassurance is required. I do not prescribe topical steroids for patients with viral conjunctivitis.

Figure 35-3. Acute follicular conjunctivitis in an adult patient, with large follicles present in the inferior fornix.

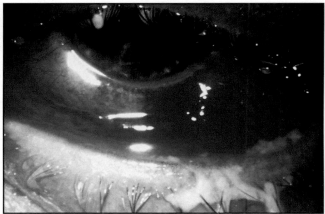

The role of topical corticosteroids remains controversial; initial symptomatic relief may occur, but sub-epithelial infiltrates with resultant visual degradation are more severe and difficult to eradicate after initial steroid therapy. Pharyngeal conjunctival fever presents acutely with follicular conjunctivitis, fever, pharyngitis, and sub-mandibular lymphadenopathy. In contrast to EKC, PCF rarely involves the cornea or forms membranes.

Primary HSV causes an acute follicular conjunctivitis with serous discharge and preauricular lymphadenopathy that is often associated with a vesicular lesion on the lid margin, fever, and upper respiratory symptoms.[1] Approximately 50% of patients have concomitant corneal epithelial punctate staining or dendrites. Treatment of HSV conjunctivitis includes topical trifluridine 1% solution 8 times per day, oral acyclovir 200 to 400 mg 5 times per day, oral valacyclovir (500 mg 2 or 3 times a day), or famciclovir (250 mg twice a day) for the prevention of corneal infection.[2]

Acute Membranous Conjunctivitis

The etiology of acute membranous or pseudomembranous conjunctivitis may be elusive and require cultures be obtained.[1] Common causes include EKC, HSV, B-hemolytic streptococci, S. aureus, and rarely C. diphtheriae.

As discussed, being able to classify the type of conjunctivitis is essential in determining the etiology, directing the necessary laboratory workup, and tailoring therapy.

References

1. Krachmer JH, Mannis MJ, Holland EJ. *Cornea, Volume 1: Fundamentals, Diagnosis and Management.* 2nd ed. Philadelphia, PA: Mosby; 2005.
2. American Academy of Ophthalmology Cornea/External Disease Panel, Preferred Practice Patterns Committee. *Conjunctivitis.* San Francisco, CA: American Academy of Ophthalmology; 2008.
3. Sheikh A, Hurwitz B. Antibiotics versus placebo for acute bacterial conjunctivitis. *Cochrane Database Syst Rev.* 2006;19(2):CD001211.
4. Ullman S, Roussel TJ, Forster RK. Gonococcal keratoconjunctivitis. *Surv Ophthalmol.* 1987;32(3):199-208.

SECTION IV

CONTACT LENSES

36

My Patient Complains of Redness and Photophobia After Sleeping With Contact Lenses. The Exam Shows Diffuse Patchy Epithelial and Anterior Stromal Infiltrates. What Should I Do?

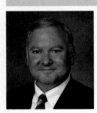

Stephen C. Kaufman, MD, PhD

White-gray corneal infiltrates are a common complication associated with contact lens wear. Although infectious keratitis is a very serious problem, contact lens-associated sterile corneal infiltrates are a more common finding. Initially, it is difficult to clinically differentiate between the infiltrates associated with a noninfectious and infectious keratitis. The infiltrates appear as single or multiple white to white-gray lesions, and they are located in the subepithelial region of the cornea. They are commonly associated with surrounding edema and inflammation. Conjunctival injection is also a common finding. The patient typically experiences pain and photophobia.

This case scenario is not uncommon. Our young patient wore her lenses overnight and now has a corneal infiltrate, conjunctival hyperemia, and discomfort (Figure 36-1). It is significant to note that she was presumably healthy up to this point, but the clinician must specifically ask the patient about her general health and ocular history. Also, on slit-lamp examination, the corneal epithelium was intact. It would be important to ask whether the patient awoke with pain or whether her pain was associated with some later event, such as attempted contact lens hydration, lens removal, or replacement.

Figure 36-1. The patient slept in her contact lenses and now has a corneal infiltrate, hyperemic conjunctiva, and pain.

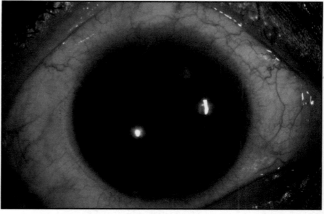

Management

Because the patient experienced the pain upon waking with the contact lenses in her eyes, and because the corneal epithelium was intact, it was much more likely that this is a case of noninfectious keratitis. This type of clinical presentation results from inflammation and corneal edema secondary to hypoxia, which is also occasionally associated with "tight-lens" syndrome.[1] Therefore, initially, I do not typically scrape and culture these corneas. I commonly treat these cases with preservative-free artificial tears and a mild steroid, such as fluorometholone or loteprednol 2 to 4 times daily for 3 to 7 days. However, because of the ever-present risk that this could be the result of an infectious etiology, it is quite reasonable to add an epithelium-friendly, broad-spectrum antibiotic such as a topical later-generation fluoroquinolone. The patient must understand that she is required to contact the clinician if her symptoms worsen, and she should be seen in 1 or 2 days after the initiation of treatment. Although her signs and symptoms may not have completely resolved in 1 or 2 days, they should be improved. If not, the steroids must be stopped, and the area of the infiltrates must be cultured. I will also begin fortified vancomycin (50 mg/mL) and tobramycin (15 mg/mL). Some clinicians also culture the contact lenses and the contact lens case, but many contact lens cases are contaminated by organisms that are not the same organisms found in corneal cultures.[2] Any history of possible ocular herpes virus infection should be investigated. If there is any history of swimming with soft contact lenses in place, we will also get cultures for acanthamoeba and perform confocal microscopy. However, I believe that this is somewhat unique and regional.

If the patient had noted that the pain did not begin until she attempted to hydrate the lens, remove the lens, or replace the lens, then I would consider either a toxic reaction from use of an incorrect eye drop or solution or incomplete rinsing of the lenses. The reaction to toxic substances in the eye or a hypersensitivity reaction can result in corneal infiltrates, a nummular keratitis, and possibly corneal edema but there is frequently an area of punctate epithethelial keratopathy (PEK) present, which this patient did not exhibit.[3]

Mechanical trauma associated with the removal of a dry lens that was left on the eye overnight or scratching the ocular surface during lens removal can cause eye pain, but slit-lamp examination would reveal corneal or conjunctival epithelial defects, which are not typically associated with an infiltrate, after just 1 night.

There are exceptions to these general guidelines, but the clinician can use the history and examination to form a revised differential diagnosis list and treatment plan. For example, did the patient come into contact with someone who had an adenovirus conjunctivitis ("pink eye"), and does she have conjunctival follicles and a pre-auricular node?

If the superior limbus and superior bulbar conjunctiva are the predominantly affected sites, then a diagnosis of contact lens-related superior limbal keratoconjunctivitis (SLK) could be entertained. Unlike the more common SLK, contact lens-related SLK is not associated with thyroid abnormalities, but it can result in pain, photophobia, and possible PEK.

Have these symptoms been present longer than a day? If so, an infectious keratitis would be more strongly considered in the differential diagnosis list. Is there a purulent discharge and epithelial defect, which is commonly associated with a bacterial keratitis? Despite the absence of a purulent discharge, a bacterial keratitis should always be considered. Antibiotic therapy should be tailored to your region, with coverage of *Pseudomonas*, which is a very common contact lens-related pathogen, and combined with close follow-up examinations.[4]

Does the patient swim with her contact lenses in place, or does she use tap water to soak her soft contact lenses? Is the patient's pain greater than expected considering the corneal appearance, and is there a fine stippling of the corneal epithelium (Figure 36-2)? These are early signs of an amoebic keratitis, which we examine by confocal microscopy (Figure 36-3), culture, and by removal of the entire area of affected epithelium in an attempt to eliminate as many organisms as possible. We start anti-amoebic therapy then. Other findings such as ring infiltrates and neurokeratitis are later ocular findings associated with an amoebic keratitis.

Are there satellite lesions (white spots) associated with the infiltrate, which may portend the presence of a fungal keratitis? We will also perform confocal microscopy if a fungal keratitis is suspected. The use of a specific contact lens solution was recently associated with an increase in fungal keratitis. The solution was removed from the market, but some patients had purchased a large supply of the solution and continued to use it after the recall. This illustrates the importance of constantly keeping current by reviewing the ophthalmic literature and participating in ophthalmic forums.

Summary

Contact lens type; lens care; the number of hours of contact lens wear per day; and the presence of dry eyes, blepharitis, and other ocular conditions can also increase the risk of contact lens-associated keratitis. As always, a good history and examination will help to narrow the differential diagnosis list and guide treatment.

Figure 36-2. This patient swims in lakes with her contact lenses in place. In this eye with early acanthamoeba keratitis, a patchy, stippled corneal epithelium is seen with a faint infiltrate adjacent to a corneal nerve.

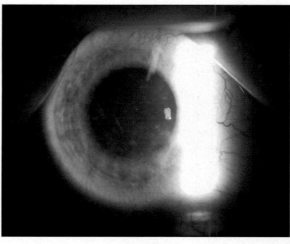

Figure 36-3. This confocal photomicrograph demonstrates an acanthamoeba cyst within the corneal stroma (arrowhead). The size is approximately 45 μm in diameter.

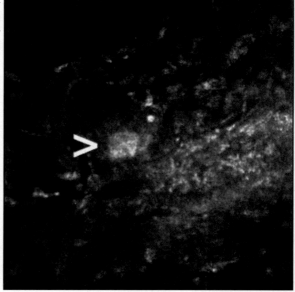

References

1. Kaufman SC, Dabezies OH, Klyce SD, et al. Corneal changes from contact lenses. In: Kaufman HE, Barron BA, McDonald MB, Kaufman SC, eds. *Companion Handbook to the Cornea*. 3rd ed. Boston, MA: Butterworth-Heinemann; 2000:661-680.
2. Krachmer JH, Purcell JJ Jr. Bacterial corneal ulcers in cosmetic soft contact lens wearers. *Arch Ophthalmol.* 1978;96(1):57-61.
3. Morgan JF. Complications associated with contact lens solutions. *Ophthalmology.* 1979;86(6):1107-1119.
4. Dart JK, Stapleton F, Minassian D. Contact lenses and other risk factors in microbial keratitis. *Lancet.* 1991;338 (8768):650-653.

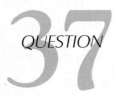

A Young Patient Has Best Spectacle-Corrected Visual Acuity of 20/30 OD and 20/25 OS, and Retinoscopy Shows Scissor Reflex. Is This Keratoconus?

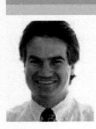

Yaron S. Rabinowitz, MD

In this instance, I would do a hard contact lens over-refraction and carefully examine this patient's corneal topography. If the hard contact lens over-refraction gets the patient to 20/20 in each eye and the corneal topography (sagittal) shows a pattern of inferior steepening with skewed steep radial axes above and below the horizontal meridian, the diagnosis is clear cut—this is a case of "early" keratoconus.

If this patient only had inferior steepening on corneal topography and uncorrected vision of 20/20, this presents a different diagnostic dilemma. To assist surgeons with the diagnostic challenge in such patients, I suggest physicians use a classification scheme for keratoconus based on videokeratography and clinical signs, which we recently published[1]:

1. Clinical keratoconus—slit-lamp signs of keratoconus: Stromal thinning with or without Vogt's striae, a Fleischer ring, superficial scarring, Munson's sign accompanied by scissoring of the red reflex on dilated retinoscopy, and an asymmetric bowtie with skewed radial axis (AB/SRAX) pattern on videokeratography

2. "Early" keratoconus: No slit-lamp findings but scissoring on dilated retinoscopy accompanied by an AB/SRAX pattern on videokeratography (Figure 37-1)

3. "Forme fruste" keratoconus: No slit-lamp findings, no scissoring on retinoscopy, and an AB/SRAX pattern[2,3]

4. Keratoconus "suspect": No slit-lamp findings, no scissoring on retinoscopy, and a pattern of inferior steepening on corneal topography only

Figure 37-1. Early keratoconus demonstrating an AB/SRAX pattern.

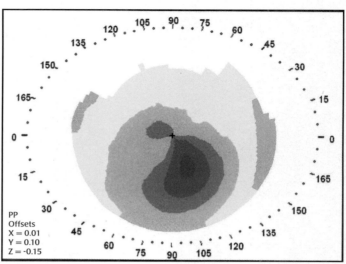

The problem posed as a question, therefore, clearly falls into category 2, and treatment options can then be tailored to this patient (see discussion to follow). Keratoconus "suspect" is more commonly the diagnostic dilemma. The following issues need to be kept in mind to determine whether such a patient is at high risk for developing keratoconus:

* A family history of keratoconus
* A history of progressive change in refraction
* Artifacts inducing inferior steepening (ie, dry eye, inferior lid compression, contact lens warpage, previous injury, or scarring of the eye)
* Inferior steepening as a variation of normal. In a published article by our group,[4] we demonstrated that up to 19% of normal patients could have patterns with inferior steepening on corneal topography, while 0.5% had an AB/SRAX pattern. In cases of inferior steepening, which represent a diagnostic dilemma, the following adjunctive tests may be useful:
  + Calculation of the I-S value: Any values greater than 3 standard deviations[5] of normal should be carefully re-examined, remembering that different topographers have different proprietary algorithms so you cannot necessarily transpose from one topographer to the next
  + Cornea OCT is very helpful (ie, if an area of inferior steepening is accompanied by thinning of the cornea on OCT, this eye should be regarded as highly suspicious)
  + The Pentacam may also demonstrate areas of corneal thinning where the axial topography shows elevation or steepening on topography
  + An abnormal float on Orbscan for those who have that device could be factored into the overall evaluation, although it is my opinion that a combination of saggital topography and OCT is all that is required for modern-day diagnosis or refractive surgery screening to rule out suspicious corneas (Figure 37-2)

The differential diagnosis of keratoconus should include pellucid marginal degeneration, Terrien's marginal degeneration, keratoglobus, and other causes of corneal thinning,

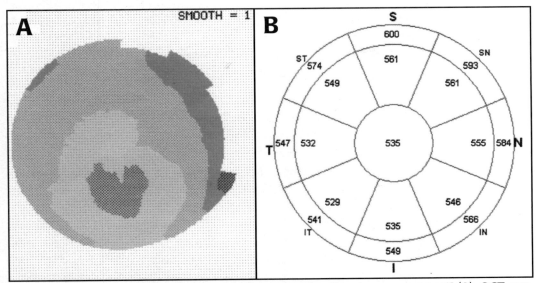

Figure 37-2. Inferior steepening on corneal topography; "keratoconus suspect" (A). OCT confirms the presence of corneal thinning in the steep area on topography (B).

such as chronic inflammations. These can be differentiated from keratoconus on clinical evaluation and corneal topography. There is a high association of allergy and atopic conjunctivitis in patients with keratoconus, and, as such, many of them are eye rubbers. While the role of eye rubbing in the pathogenesis of keratoconus remains a cause for debate, it is reasonable to suggest to patients with keratoconus not to rub their eyes as this may play a role in the progression of the disease.

Treatment Options

A minority of patients with keratoconus can be managed with either glasses or soft contact lenses in mild forms of the disease. The vast majority of patients need rigid contact lenses to gain crisp visual acuity. For patients with good visual acuity and who tolerate their contact lenses well, no further treatment is required.

In patients who are contact lens intolerant and who have K readings of 58 D or less, Intacs or intracorneal ring segments are good options. This will flatten the cornea and improve contact lens tolerance. In many instances, this surgical procedure also has secondary benefits (ie, improving both the uncorrected and corrected visual acuity). It does this by decreasing the higher-order aberrations of the cornea.[6] In patients who are highly myopic and further want to decrease their dependence on glasses or contact lenses, a phakic IOL (Visian ICL or Verisyse) could be considered, in particular the toric versions, which unfortunately are currently only available outside of the United States.

For patients with advanced disease and who are contact lens intolerant or have central scarring with poor acuity, corneal transplants are the most viable treatment option. In many parts of the world, lamellar transplants are offered; however, in my experience, while this decreases the risk of rejection, these patients do not have good quality visual acuity following their procedures. My preference is to perform full-thickness penetrating keratoplasties with the Intralase laser (IEK—Intralase enabled keratoplasty). The procedure is quick (less than 45 minutes), is safer, results in less postoperative astigmatism, and provides a large wound surface area, which results in much quicker and stronger wound healing. Patients can then have any residual astigmatism corrected with contact lenses, LASIK, or PRK with mitomycin C.

In patients whose disease is rapidly progressive and whose corneas are thicker than 400 µm, collagen crosslinking is a new treatment option that is currently being investigated. There has been significant experience in Europe, and clinical trials in the United States are currently underway. Initial reports suggest that this treatment is safe, and it does appear to have an effect on the progression, although with currently available data, this is difficult to prove. Our center is currently conducting a clinical trial comparing crosslinking to a combination of Intacs and crosslinking.

PRK in patients with keratoconus is a controversial treatment because there is always the potential for progressive corneal thinning or thinning the cornea too much with untoward outcomes. It is reasonable, however, to treat mild cases with PRK and mitomycin with the correct informed consent, and our group has been doing this for many years with good success. Combining this procedure with collagen crosslinking may add a level of safety, and new algorithms available on excimer lasers with topographically guided software may improve outcomes. A combination of Intacs and PRK with mitomycin can also be used in select cases with good results.

References

1. Li X, Yang H, Rabinowitz YS. Keratoconus: classification scheme based on videokeratography and clinical signs. *J Cataract Refract Surgery.* 2009;35(9):1597-1603.
2. Amsler M. Early diagnosis and microsymptoms. *Ophthalmologica.* 1965;149(5):438-446.
3. Li X, Rabinowitz YS, Rasheed K, Yang H. Longitudinal study of the normal eyes in unilateral keratoconus patients. *Ophthalmology.* 2004;111(3):440-446.
4. Rabinowitz YS, Yang H, Brickman Y, et al. Videokeratography database of normal human corneas. *Br J Ophthalmol.* 1996;80(7):610-616.
5. Rabinowitz YS. Videokeratographic indices to aid in screening for keratoconus. *J Refract Surg.* 1995;11(5):371-379.
6. Rabinowitz YS, Li X, Ignacio TS, Maguen E. INTACS inserts using the femtosecond laser compared to the mechanical spreader in the treatment of keratoconus. *J Refract Surg.* 2006;22(8):764-771.

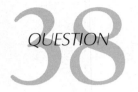

WHAT SHOULD I DO FOR A PATIENT WHO WEARS SOFT CONTACT LENSES AND COMPLAINS OF DRY AND ITCHY EYES?

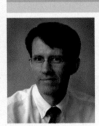

Thomas F. Mauger, MD

A careful history is often the key to the successful diagnosis and management of these patients. It should be focused on the onset of the symptoms in relation to the contact lens wear as well as other compounding conditions (Table 38-1). A history of contact lens wear should include the type of contact lenses, wearing time, and solution use. The patient should also be questioned as to his or her wearing time and areas of noncompliance, including overnight wear or unapproved liquids to wet contact lenses such as water. When scheduling his or her appointment, he or she should be told to bring his or her contact lenses, contact lens case(s), and solutions.

Also, ask about underlying ocular problems such as a history of herpes simplex keratitis, previously treated conjunctivitis, dry eye, rosacea, or the use of one of many systemic medications that can reduce tear production. Symptoms of primary or secondary Sjogren's syndrome should be explored and laboratory and rheumatologic workup pursued when appropriate.

Examination

A careful external and slit-lamp examination should focus on the contact lens on the eye, the contact lens case, the eyelids, conjunctiva, limbus, and cornea along with a complete ocular examination. The principal areas of concern are listed in Table 38-2.

Table 38-1
History

- Are the symptoms relieved with cessation of contact lens wear?
- Type of contact lenses, solutions, and care regimen including use of water
- Wearing schedule, overnight use
- Seasonal variation in symptoms
- Time of day of symptoms
- History of ocular problems: Herpes simplex keratitis, recurrent conjunctivitis, rosacea, dry eye, Sjogen's syndrome
- Medication history

Table 38-2
Examination

- External exam—lid function, signs of Rosacea
- Evaluate contact lens fit and protein deposits
- Examination of the contact lens case for overall condition and presence of a biofilm
- Lid margins, tarsal conjunctiva

Differential Diagnosis

The most likely etiologies of dry, itchy eyes in a contact lens wearer are underlying dry eye, blepharitis, giant papillary conjunctivitis (GPC), hypersensitivity reaction, or allergic conjunctivitis further exacerbated by the wear of the contact lens.

Contact lenses and solutions can lead to toxic corneal changes. These can include conjunctivitis and also corneal epitheliopathies (Figure 38-1). Decreasing wearing time, changing solutions, or changing to daily disposable contact lenses may be indicated.

Dry eye is a very common cause of contact lens-related irritation in middle age or older patients and may preclude the comfortable wearing of contact lenses. Contact lenses alter the precorneal tear film, which may worsen or improve the symptoms of dry eye.[1] If contact lens wear is an exacerbating factor, a change in the contact lens, solution, or wearing time can sometimes be helpful. In addition to topical lubrication, punctal occlusion may be helpful. Topical cyclosporine (Restasis, Allergan, Irvine, CA) can improve tear production as well as reduce ocular surface inflammation over time, but requires several months of treatment in most cases. Contact lenses should be removed prior to instilling Restasis. Elimination of confounding systemic medications that reduce tear production is also helpful.

Symptomatic blepharitis is quite common with or without rosacea as an undiagnosed cause of ocular irritation and contact lens intolerance in a corneal referral practice. It frequently occurs concurrently with dry eye. The treatment of this may include local

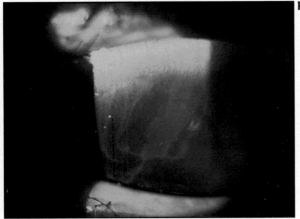

Figure 38-1. Toxic corneal epitheliopathy.

mechanical cleaning of the lid margins as well as antibiotic ointment to the lid margins to reduce the bacterial load. Topical steroid drops or ointments may be helpful in the initial treatment phase to give rapid reduction of inflammation. The treatment of rosacea-related blepharoconjunctivitis may be managed with the use of systemic tetracycline derivatives.

Giant papillary conjunctivitis is related to a combination of mechanical irritation from the edge and surface of a contact lens (or other foreign body) and the protein deposits on the surface of the contact lens.[2] Topical steroids, nonsteroidal anti-inflammatory drugs (NSAIDs), and mast cell stabilizers may be used, but they are often ineffective. Trials of alternate contact lenses and solutions may be helpful. Disposable contact lenses eliminate protein deposits and solution reactions as possible causes. Reduction of wearing time will usually decrease the symptoms. In recalcitrant cases, cessation of contact lens wear either temporarily or permanently may be necessary. The papilla may take months to resolve after cessation of the contact lens wear.

Allergic conjunctivitis may be seasonal and can be controlled with systemic and/or topical antihistamines, topical mast cell stabilizers, and NSAIDs. Topical steroids may be required for more severe vernal conjunctivitis. Contact lens wear may be difficult during these periods. Avoidance, if possible, of the inciting agent is an integral part of therapy. If the inciting agent cannot be easily deduced, allergy testing by an allergist can often be helpful. Desensitization therapy can reduce the signs and symptoms of allergic conjunctivitis. Patients may develop a hypersensitivity reaction to their solutions, and switching to a hydrogen peroxide-based system or disposable contact lenses may offer relief.

Contact lens care and cleaning is critical to the prevention of more serious contact lens-related infections. The wear of contact lenses during sleep significantly increases the risk of infectious keratitis.[3] Both sterile (Figure 38-2) and infectious (Figure 38-3) keratitis may occur with prolonged contact lens wear. These are evidenced by stromal infiltration with or without overlying epithelial defect. Sterile infiltrates may be managed with topical anti-inflammatory agents; however, culturing and intensive antibiotic treatment is recommended for infectious contact lens-related keratitis.[4]

A common break in contact lens care involves the use of water in the cleaning of the contact lens case. This allows a biofilm to form that might include fungi and Acanthamoeba organisms. No current contact lens solution reliably kills Acanthamoeba.[5] The patient

Figure 38-2. Mid-peripheral contact lens-related sterile corneal infiltrate.

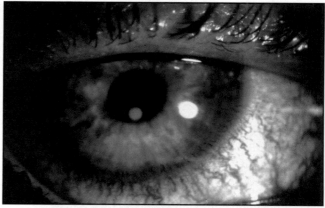

Figure 38-3. Infectious contact lens-related keratitis.

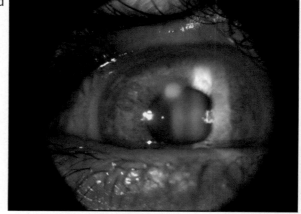

who presents with increasing ocular irritation and irregular epithelium (especially with atypical dendrites and stromal inflammation) (Figure 38-4) should have Acanthamoeba or fungal keratitis in the differential until it is ruled out. Confocal microscopy and cultures of the cornea and contact lens and case are recommended.

Summary

Contact lens wear can alter the lids, conjunctiva, and cornea. The majority of the causes of irritation can be remedied by changing the contact lens, wearing schedule, or care regimen. More serious causes can be identified through careful history and examination.

References

1. Nichols JJ, Sinnott LT. Tear film, contact lens, and patient factors associated with contact lens-related dry eye. *Invest Ophthalmol Vis Sci.* 2006;47:1319-1328.
2. Allansmith MR, Korb DR, Greiner JV, Henriquez AS, Simon MA, Finnemore VM. Giant papillary conjunctivitis in contact lens wearers. *Am J Ophthalmol.* 1977;83(5):697-708.

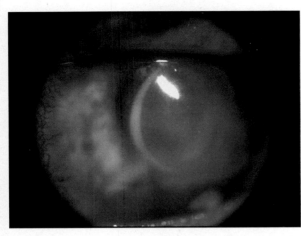

Figure 38-4. Contact lens-associated Acanthamoeba keratitis.

3. Schein OD, Buehler PO, Stamler JF, Verdier DD, Katz J. The impact of overnight wear on the risk of contact lens-associated ulcerative keratitis. *Arch Ophthalmol.* 1994;112(2):186-190.

4. Baum J, Dabezies OH Jr. Pathogenesis and treatment of "sterile" midperipheral corneal infiltrates associated with soft contact lens use. *Cornea.* 2000;19(6):777-781.

5. Shoff ME, Joslin CE, Tu EY, Kubatko L, Fuerst PA. Efficacy of contact lens systems against recent clinical and tap water Acanthamoeba isolates. *Cornea.* 2008;27(6):713-719.

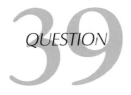

QUESTION 39

HOW SHOULD I MANAGE A PATIENT WITH KERATOCONUS WHO CANNOT TOLERATE HARD GAS-PERMEABLE CONTACT LENSES?

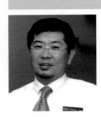

Donald Tan, FRCSG, FRCSE, FRCOphth, FAMS
(co-authored with Jod S. Mehta, BSc, MBBS, MRCOphth,
FRCOphth, FRCS(Ed))

There have been major advances in the surgical management of keratoconus in the past 2 decades. Penetrating keratoplasty had been the mainstay for treatment of advanced disease for the past 50 years, but improvements in surgical instrumentation and publication of more evidence-based comparative studies have shown equivalent visual acuity results with fewer complications with modern surgical techniques.[1]

Intra-Corneal Ring Segment

Intacs (intra-corneal ring segment) are micro-thin intra-corneal inserts made of rigid polymethylmethacrylate. They produce a flattening effect on the central cornea by effectively reducing the arc-length of the corneal lamellae. These biomechanical effects are more pronounced in thinner corneas, and they have been shown to be efficacious in patients with low to moderate keratoconus (mean K ≤ 53 D). However, in steeper corneas and hence those with more advanced keratoconus, the effect has been variable probably due to the failure of the rings to provide significant flattening effect and subsequent changes in topography. In extremely thin corneas (eg, ≤ 400 µm), there may be inadequate biomechanical rigidity of the cornea to produce an effect. There has also been higher rates of surgical complications (eg, segment exposure, extrusion), but the use of a femtosecond laser for placement of the ring segments may reduce some of the complications associated with ring segment placement in these thin corneas. More recently, groups have shown good outcomes in advanced cases.[2] The aim of ring placement in advanced cases is not to achieve uncorrected best potential vision, but to flatten the cone and improve the best spectacle-corrected visual acuity and achieve contact lens tolerance.

Radiofrequency

One study has reported the use of radiofrequency energy in the treatment of advanced keratoconus.[3] Depending on the severity of the preoperative K reading, either 8 or 16 thermal spots are applied in the 4- to 5-mm optical zone. There was a significant increase in best spectacle-corrected visual acuity at the 18-month follow-up, and all patients were able to subsequently be fitted for contact lens wear. No other studies have reported the use of this treatment in these cases.

Deep Anterior Lamellar Keratoplasty (DALK)

DALK surgery has seen a revival during the past decade, mainly due to improvements in surgical techniques. The main advantage of any anterior lamellar procedure is the preservation of the patient's own endothelium, reducing the risk of immunological allograft rejection and subsequent graft failure. The disadvantage with previous lamellar surgical techniques was the presence of stromal scarring and interface opacification from remnant host stroma remaining on Descemet's membrane (DM). Newer techniques (eg, "Big Bubble" air dissection) allow the possibility of gaining access directly to the Descemet's plane. Cleavage of the overlying stroma can be achieved by forceful air injection (as in the big bubble technique) (Figure 39-1), viscoelastic injection, or by manual dissection. Although there are few studies describing large series with this technique, evidence is now being published showing that visual acuity with these Descemet's membrane-baring techniques are equivalent to penetrating keratoplasty. However, postoperative complications were significantly less in the DALK group compared to PK.[1] The major problem with this technique is the significant learning curve in achieving big bubble formation and intraoperative microperforation with rates varying from 8% to 25%. Despite this complication occurring, one may still be able to complete the lamellar surgery without conversion to full-thickness penetrating keratoplasty with appropriate surgical maneuvers. In cases in which full baring of DM is not achieved, deep manual dissection can achieve good visual results. Due to the extra interface, they are generally poorer compared to Descemet's baring techniques. In cases following hydrops, Descemet's baring techniques may not be possible due to the risk of inadvertent splitting of DM during bubble formation. In such cases, manual dissection may be attempted, but the risk of intraoperative DM splitting is high due to the weakness of the previous rupture of DM. PK-grade tissue on standby is advised when performing such cases, but if a manual lamellar dissection is achievable, visual acuity results can be encouraging as long as the original rupture was not in the visual axis (Figure 39-2).

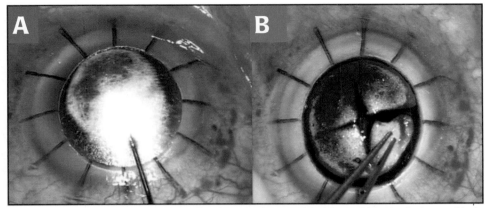

Figure 39-1. Deep anterior lamellar keratoplasty with big bubble technique. Air is injected to induce cleavage of Descemet's membrane from the overlying stroma (A). The overlying stroma is incised into 4 quadrants after big bubble formation with careful attention not to perforate Descemet's membrane (B).

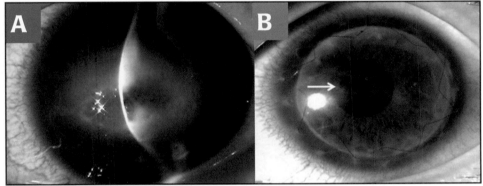

Figure 39-2. Corneal hydrops in a patient with keratoconus before (A) and after deep anterior lamellar keratoplasty (B). Note the Descemet's membrane rupture that led to hydrops is outside the visual axis (arrow).

Penetrating Keratoplasty

PK has been the definitive surgery for keratoconus during the past 50 years. Good visual outcomes are achieved in conventional PK in keratoconus cases, but as with all full-thickness procedures, long-term endothelial cell attrition will occur. This is particularly significant in patients with keratoconus who are generally young and thus require long-term corneal graft survival. In cases in which there are previous hydrops involving the visual axis, PK is the only alternative for successful visual rehabilitation. Innovative ways of performing PK have been described. Busin and colleagues described a top-hat technique in which the anterior surface of the donor button is smaller than the posterior surface.[4] This technique combined the refractive and visual outcomes of PK with the wound-healing advantage of lamellar keratoplasty. Suture removal may be performed earlier, and visual acuity results have been shown to be equivalent to conventional PK.

Mushroom keratoplasty using a large anterior surface and a smaller posterior surface has also been performed successfully in advanced keratoconus. Both of these techniques used a manual dissection method, but with the advent of the femtosecond lasers, innovative graft-host junction profiles (eg, zigzag, Christmas tree, mushroom, top hat) may be performed, significantly reducing surgical time.

Future

There has been a paradigm shift in the management of advanced keratoconus during the past 2 decades. Each case must be assessed individually, and penetrating keratoplasty can no longer be considered the first-choice procedure. The results of newer Descemet's baring techniques offer the benefits of visual acuity comparative to PK without the rates of complications. Other techniques (eg, Intacs, radiofrequency) need further investigations. Interventions aimed at reducing disease progression (eg, collagen crosslinking or keratocyte cell transplantation) may reduce the number of advanced cases in the future.

References

1. Han DC, Mehta JS, Por YM, Htoon HM, Tan DT. Comparison of outcomes of lamellar keratoplasty and penetrating keratoplasty in Keratoconus. *Am J Ophthalmol.* 2009;148(5):744-751.
2. Ertan A, Kamburoglu G. Intacs implantation using a femtosecond laser for management of keratoconus: comparison of 306 cases in different stages. *J Cataract Refract Surg.* 2008;34(9):1521-1526.
3. Lyra JM, Trindade FC, Lyra D, Bezerra A. Outcomes of radiofrequency in advanced keratoconus. *J Cataract Refract Surg.* 2007;33(7):1288-1295.
4. Busin M. A new lamellar wound configuration for penetrating keratoplasty surgery. *Arch Ophthalmol.* 2003;121(2):260-265.

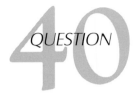
A LONG-TIME SOFT CONTACT LENS USER COMPLAINS OF EYE IRRITATION AND HAS SUPERFICIAL PUNCTATE KERATOPATHY IN THE AREA OF CORNEAL APEX. IS THIS A POOR CONTACT LENS FIT?

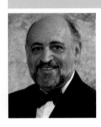

Mark J. Mannis, MD, FACS

Successful contact lens wear, be it with rigid gas-permeable, hydrophilic, or hybrid lenses, is contingent upon the dynamic relationship between the contact lens and the various components of the ocular surface. The latter include the tear film, cornea, conjunctiva, and lids, and without either a normal ocular surface or measures to manage surface abnormalities, contact lens wear will result in symptom-producing surface pathology.

Evaluation

The first step in avoiding superficial punctate keratopathy (SPK) in contact lens wear is to thoroughly evaluate the ocular surface. This should include the following:

* An evaluation of the tear film including Schirmer testing, evaluation of the tear meniscus, and tear stability (tear breakup time)
* An assessment of the lids including careful observation of evidence of anterior or posterior blepharitis as well as adequacy and rate of blinking
* Observation of the conjunctiva including the perilimbal zone, the luster of the conjunctival surface, and the pre-tarsal and forniceal conjunctiva

Assuming that these are normal, the avoidance of SPK in the contact lens wearer then hinges on the appropriate choice of lens material and the adequacy of the fit.

Management

If SPK develops in the contact lens wearer, I use the following decision tree:

* In the presence of anterior or posterior blepharitis:

  + Initiate lid hygiene, including effective lid scrubs
  + If indicated, consider a course of oral doxycycline

* In the presence of a decreased tear meniscus, mucus in the pre-corneal tear film, a diminished Schirmer test, or a decreased tear breakup time:

  + Initiate artificial tears
  + Consider punctal occlusion
  + Consider initiating topical cyclosporine

* In the presence of evidence of limbal disease (ie, epithelial streaming, vascularization of the limbus), consider the following:

  + Altering contact lens material
  + Decreasing wear time
  + Discontinuing CL wear temporarily or permanently

Case Studies

The following examples are cases in which the variants of SPK are dependent on either the contact lens/cornea relationship or ocular surface pathology that results in lens-induced ocular surface disease:

* This patient wore rigid gas-permeable lenses for vision correction in keratoconus and developed symptoms of discomfort and blurring after several hours of lens wear (Figure 40-1).

  Diagnosis: punctate keratopathy secondary to tight lens syndrome.

  Treatment: contact lens re-fit with a flatter base curve.

Figure 40-1. Extensive punctate keratopathy in contact lens wearer with keratoconus resulting from a tightly fit contact lens. Note the impression of the tight lens in the periphery of the cornea with fluorescein pooling.

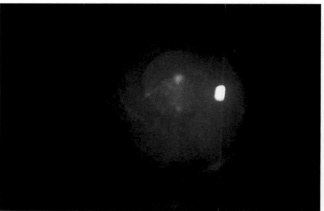

✳ This patient complained of burning and decreased vision while wearing hydrophilic lenses for 10 to 12 hours daily. The tear meniscus was markedly diminished, and the Schirmer test was 5 mm (with anesthetic). The predominant pattern was inferior distribution of the punctate keratopathy (Figure 40-2).

Diagnosis: tear film insufficiency.

Treatment: non-preserved artificial tears, temporary punctal occlusion, and re-fit with a low water content lens material. The lower water content lens is less likely to "steal" aqueous tears from the ocular surface.

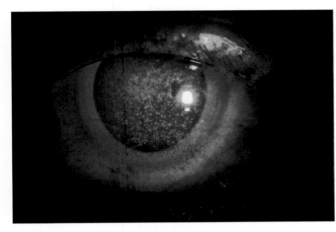

Figure 40-2. Diffuse, predominantly inferiorly distributed, coarse punctate keratopathy in a soft lens wearer with insufficient tear film.

✳ A 42-year-old patient wearing daily-wear contact lenses developed burning and foreign body sensation shortly after inserting lenses. Examination revealed lid margins (Figure 40-3).

Diagnosis: chronic meibomian dysfunction with tear film instability.

Treatment: contact lens wear was discontinued for 1 month, during which time the patient was treated with a course of doxycycline and intensive lid hygiene. Lens wear was renewed successfully with continued regular lid hygiene.

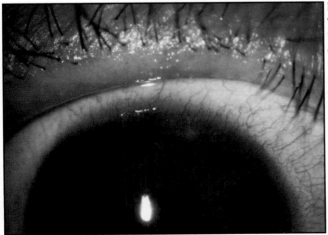

Figure 40-3. Lid margins consistent with chronic blepharitis including meibomian gland inspissation, collarettes, lid margin inflammation, lash irregularity, and peripheral corneal scarring and vascularization consistent with chronic inflammatory disease.

* This 46-year-old woman wore contact lenses on a continuous-wear basis for 10 years. She slept with the lenses in place, removing them briefly for cleaning only every 2 weeks. She presented with decreased vision and discomfort after wearing the lenses for several hours. The corneal staining pattern appeared as in Figure 40-4. Diagnosis: contact lens-induced limbal stem cell dysfunction.

Treatment: based on the assessment of significant contact lens damage to the limbus, lens wear was discontinued for 6 months, and the patient was treated with lubricants and spectacles. The patient desired to be re-fit for lenses. Loosely fit, high water content soft lenses were fit for daily wear only.

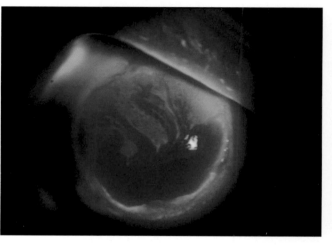

Figure 40-4. Characteristic "streaming" epithelial keratopathy consistent with localized stem cell depletion from chronic hydrophilic contact lens wear. (Photograph courtesy of Ivan R. Schwab, MD, University of California, Davis).

Summary

The accurate diagnosis and management of SPK in conjunction with contact lenses depends on a thorough examination of the cornea for the pattern of staining as well as an assessment of the ocular adnexa. I look very carefully at both the pattern and the distribution of staining, which will often pinpoint the diagnosis. It is equally important to examine the ocular adnexa critically. In general, treatment of contact lens-induced SPK will include optimization of both the tear film, the lid margins, and the specific materials used and parameters of the contact lens fit.

Recommended Readings

Mannis MJ, Zadnik K, Coral-Ghanem C, Kara-José N. *Contact Lenses in Ophthalmic Practice*. New York, NY: Springer; 2004.

Silbert JA. *Anterior Segment Complications of Contact Lens Wear*. New York, NY: Churchill Livingstone; 1994.

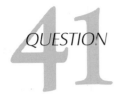

41

A LONG-TIME SOFT CONTACT LENS USER COMPLAINS OF EYE IRRITATION AND HAS SUPERFICIAL PUNCTATE KERATOPATHY IN THE SUPERIOR CORNEA AND LIMBUS. WHAT SHOULD I DO?

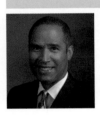

Kenneth Mark Goins, MD

In the setting of limbal stem cell deficiency (LSCD), a patient may present with either acute or chronic eye pain and photophobia from recurrent corneal erosion and persistent epithelial defect, pannus formation with associated corneal neovascularization, and loss of corneal clarity due to conjunctivalization of the surface. With respect to severity of disease, LSCD may be diffuse or focal. One or both eyes may be involved depending on the etiology of disease.

Examination Findings

There may be a history of excessive contact lens wearing time. Visual acuity may range from 20/20 to counting fingers, with worse acuity associated with visual axis involvement. Slit-lamp examination usually shows a whorled haze to the ocular surface. Application of Rose Bengal to the ocular surface may show staining on the surface epithelium, suggestive of the presence of abnormal limbal stem cell maturation and keratinization (Figure 41-1). Because conjunctival surface epithelium is more permeable to fluorescein, there may be increased intracellular uptake without the presence of an epithelial defect (Figure 41-2). All of these findings are suggestive of an abnormality in the limbal stem cell maturation process. Impression cytology may then be used to determine the presence of cytokeratin type 19 cells, which would confirm the suspicion of LSCD.[1] Confocal microscopy may also be used to diagnose early surface conjunctivalization associated with LSCD.

Figure 41-1. This is a slit-lamp photograph of a contact lens patient with early LSCD. There is a superior pannus present at 12 o'clock. A whorl-like haze can be seen within the epithelium of the visual axis. Rose Bengal has been applied to the ocular surface, and there is mild uptake along the corneal surface cells at 12 and 6 o'clock.

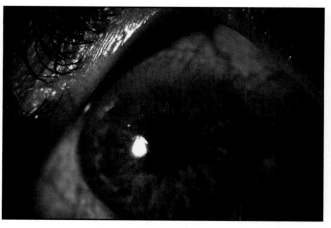

Figure 41-2. In the same patient, fluorescein has been applied to the ocular surface. The fluorescein is readily permeable to the dye at 12 and 6 o'clock, confirming the suspicion of LSCD from conjunctivalization.

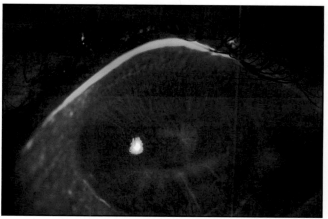

Differential Diagnosis

On initial presentation, the diagnosis may not be readily apparent. Epithelial herpes simplex virus (HSV) keratitis and acanthamoeba keratitis should be in the differential diagnosis. Corneal cultures (ie, bacteria, fungal, viral), PCR testing (HSV and acanthamoeba), and confocal microscopic examination for infectious pathogens should be considered.

Treatment Plan

REMOVAL OF THE CONTACT LENS

In the setting of contact lens-related LSCD, the first line of treatment is to remove the offending agent. A contact lens holiday is in order to allow the recovery of limbal stem cell function. As a conservative estimate, attempting to resume contact lens wear prior to 3 to 6 months of rest may prolong the duration of disease and worsen vision. If the contact lens solution (ie, preservative) is felt to be the main cause, use of a soft daily-wear disposable contact lens may provide an adequate wearing time with no further increase in limbal toxicity.

MANAGEMENT OF THE OCULAR SURFACE

Concomitant keratoconjunctivitis sicca must be managed. It is not uncommon for the chronic contact lens patient to have a reduction in corneal sensation and a resultant neurotrophic keratopathy. If the Schirmer's test is reduced, punctal occlusion is recommended to provide a larger aqueous layer of tears. Topical cyclosporine A 0.05% to 2% may be used twice daily to increase the production of the aqueous portion of the tear film. It may also have an immunologic protective effect on the activated T-cell lymphocyte destruction of accessory lacrimal gland and goblet cells, which may occur in preservative allergy. Twenty percent autologous serum eye drops may provide additional growth factors, insulin, and neurotransmitters (ie, substance P), which may improve surface epithelialization.

REDUCTION OF CORNEAL NEOVASCULARIZATION

Topical corticosteroids used 2 to 4 times daily may reduce pannus formation, inhibit the attraction of immune cells to the region, and improve vision and comfort. Long-term use may be necessary depending upon the extent of disease. Topical bevacizumab (Avastin) 5 mg/mL, an anti-vascular endothelial growth factor (VEGF) antibody, may be used up to 4 times daily for recalcitrant cases. Long-term topical use of bevacizumab is not recommended due to the risk of neurotrophic keratopathy and corneal thinning. If corneal neovascularization is associated with melting, the addition of topical medroxyprogesterone 1% (Provera) drops 2 to 4 times daily may be beneficial in reversing the inflammatory process.

RECALCITRANT CASES

For contact lens-related LSCD, which is progressive and associated with loss of corneal clarity, surgical intervention is often necessary. For focal LSCD, amniotic membrane transplantation may be used to reduce inflammation, inhibit neovascularization, and promote epithelialization. For diffuse LSCD, if there is no involvement of the contralateral eye, autologous limbal stem cell transplantation is the preferred modality of treatment.[2,3] In the setting of bilateral LSCD, keratolimbal allograft with systemic immunosuppression is the most common intervention used today.[4]

Summary

LSCD associated with contact lens wear may result in significant vision loss. Early diagnosis and medical treatment is often safe and effective. In recalcitrant cases, surgical intervention with AMT and/or KLAL can restore a normal ocular surface and vision.

References

1. Donisi PM, Rama P, Fasolo A, Ponzin D. Analysis of limbal stem cell deficiency by corneal impression cytology. *Cornea*. 2003;22(6):533-538.
2. Kenyon KR, Tseng SC. Limbal autograft transplantation for ocular surface disorders. *Ophthalmology*. 1989;96(5):709-722.

3. Clinch TE, Goins KM, Cobo LM. Treatment of contact lens related ocular surface disorders with autologous conjunctival transplantation. *Ophthalmology.* 1992;99(4):634-638.

4. Cauchi PA, Ang GS, Azuara-Blanco A, Burr JM. A systematic literature review of surgical interventions for limbal stem cell deficiency in humans. *Am J Ophthalmol.* 2008;146(2):251-259.

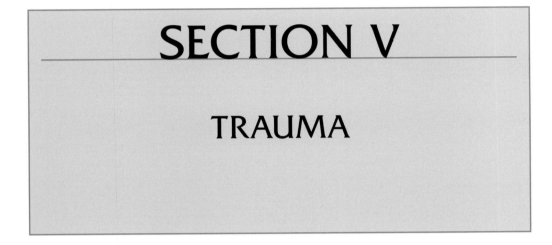

SECTION V

TRAUMA

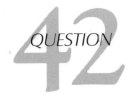

42

A Piece of Glass Flew Into My Patient's Eye. The Exam Shows Central Corneal Perforation <1 mm in Diameter. The Anterior Chamber is Shallow, but Formed. How Should I Close This Wound?

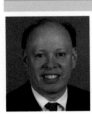

Roberto Pineda, MD

This patient has suffered a perforating corneal injury from a projectile object. A careful history is mandatory but often difficult if the patient was chemically impaired at the time of injury or if the patient is a child. In such cases, it is prudent to obtain imaging studies of the eye and orbit. If suspicion is very low or more advanced imaging modalities are not available, plain film radiography may be all that is required. However, nonmetallic foreign bodies such as glass are not easily seen on plain X-ray films and may be missed. Computed tomography is now the standard diagnostic test for imaging the traumatized eye and orbit and is available in most hospitals. Current-generation computed tomographic machines can detect nonmetallic radiolucent foreign bodies 1 mm in size. A CT scan of eye and orbit is suggested with both axial and coronal sections (1-mm sections). MR imaging may detect and localize a small nonmetallic foreign body such as glass with an image quality superior to that provided by CT for soft tissues and nonmagnetic IOFBs, but this takes longer, is less available, and is more expensive.

In addition to the slit-lamp exam, the pupil should be dilated so that the fundus can be examined. Careful examination of the periocular tissue is also warranted to rule out other sites of penetration from foreign body material. Seidel testing of the corneal wound is necessary to help determine the best options for closing the wound (Figures 42-1A and 1B). Prophylactic antibiotics (oral or IV) are mandated in all cases of ocular perforation.

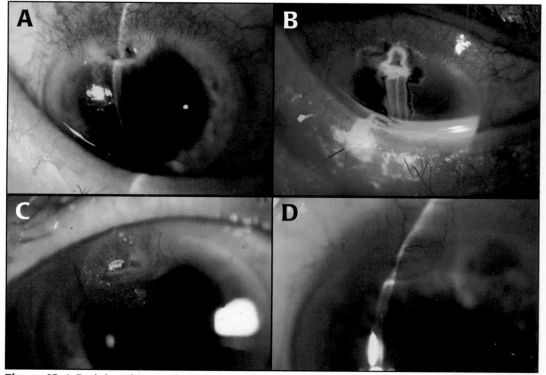

Figure 42-1. Peripheral corneal ulceration with perforation (A). Seidel positive corneal ulceration (B). Corneal perforation 1 month after application of glue (C). Area of perforation after removal of glue with wound healing (D). (Photos courtesy of Jonathan Primack, MD. Reprinted with permission.)

Treatment

Depending on Seidel testing results, different approaches can be employed to close the 1-mm perforation. If the wound is self-sealing and relatively clean with little debris, placement of an extended-wear therapeutic soft contact lens and aqueous suppression (topical beta-blocker or alpha-agonist) may be adequate for wound closure, allowing the anterior chamber to reform. An eye shield or glasses should be worn to avoid inadvertent touching of the cornea. The contact lens is usually left in place for several weeks with topical antibiotics and a mild steroid. This approach is particularly beneficial when the perforation involves the visual axis as in this case because unlike glue, it does not interfere with vision. Avoiding closure of the wound with sutures eliminates additional scarring and astigmatism. However, many times, the perforation is not self-sealing and surgical closure of the wound is required.

The use of tissue adhesives is an effective means of addressing small corneal perforations and has been used for defects of up to 2 mm. The application of cyanoacrylate glue is a simple in-office or minor surgery procedure used to close this type of defect.[1] Several brands of medical grade isobutyl-2-cyanoacrylate glue have been used, such as Dermabond. Commercial glues, such as Superglue, are methyl-2-cyanoacrylate and should be avoided as they result in secondary irritation due to formaldehyde released into the tear film during polymer breakdown.[2]

For this patient, it is easiest to glue the perforation while the patient is lying down under a microscope. However, adhesive application may be possible at the slit lamp as well. Topical anesthesia and a lid speculum are employed. Formal prepping of the eye is usually not necessary. However, epithelium around the perforation needs to be removed (1 to 2 mm) in order for the glue to adhere. Application of glue over epithelium will result in loss of the polymerized glue plug within a day or 2 of application as the corneal epithelium sloughs off. Although not mentioned in this scenario, if iris is plugging the wound, consider filtered air or light use of a viscoelastic to displace the iris before applying the glue. Attempt to dry the stromal bed as much as possible before application. Very importantly, avoid excessive glue as it irritates the eye, often results in early expulsion of glue, and limits examination of the treated area.

Application of the glue may be performed in many ways, including directly to the cornea, through the use of a microapplicator (with glue) or microtip (27- or 30-gauge needle), or via a blunt side of a cellulose spear or plastic disc (2 to 3 mm) attached to a wooden applicator for 30 seconds (polymerization is enhanced by the presence of OH$^-$ anions, abundant in aqueous and water) (Figures 42-1C and 1D).

If glue is not available or cannot effectively seal the corneal perforation, suturing the perforation is always an option. With a central corneal perforation, consider 11-0 nylon to minimize scarring, and use as few sutures as possible. 10-0 nylon is acceptable if 11-0 nylon is not available. If the wound continues to leak, consider the addition of glue and/or a therapeutic contact lens.

Last, with irregular central corneal perforations that do not close with a few simple sutures, or if there are issues with cyanoacrylate glue and long-term contact lenses, several layers of amniotic membrane can be used to close a small corneal perforation. This can be combined with the use of a fibrin-thrombin tissue adhesive such as Tisseal to avoid sutures and, therefore, scarring.

References

1. Vote BJ, Elder MJ. Cyanoacrylate glue for corneal perforations: a description of a surgical technique and a review of the literature. *Clin Experiment Ophthalmol.* 2000;28(6):437-442.
2. Chan SM, Boisjoly H. Advances in the use of adhesives in ophthalmology. *Curr Opin Ophthalmol.* 2004;15(4):305-310.

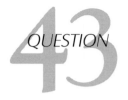
MY PATIENT WAS SPLASHED WITH CEMENT IN BOTH EYES. HE HAS RED, IRRITATED EYES AND BLURRY VISION. THE EXAM SHOWS DEBRIS ON THE CONJUNCTIVA AND UNDER THE LIDS, DIFFUSE SPK IN THE RIGHT EYE, AND CENTRAL CORNEAL EPITHELIAL DEFECT IN THE LEFT EYE. WHAT SHOULD I WATCH FOR?

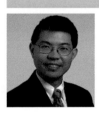

Bennie H. Jeng, MD

The spectrum of chemical burns to the eye is very broad, ranging from mild epithelial disruption to severe ocular and intraocular damage. While acid burns can cause severe destruction of the ocular surface, alkali burns can be even more destructive because saponification of cell membranes can lead to rapid penetration of the alkali through the cornea and sclera into the eye, causing destruction of intraocular contents. Although the prognosis of the injured eye depends on the extent of the injury, it also depends on the rapidity of and modalities of treatment. Thus, all chemical burns to the eye, no matter how seemingly minor, must be treated immediately as the extent of ocular surface damage can be severe depending on the chemical involved.

For this particular patient, if irrigation of the eyes had not yet been performed upon arrival in the office, *immediate* irrigation of both eyes must be performed, even before visual acuity is checked. Manual irrigation with saline or lactated Ringer solution with a bottle or through intravenous tubing directly into the eyes as well as upper and lower fornices should be performed. If a Morgan lens setup is available, this can be used after the initial manual irrigation; otherwise, manual irrigation should be continued. Either way, copious irrigation should be done for at least 30 minutes. Topical proparacaine drops can be useful during this process. Once this irrigation is performed, one should wait a few minutes to allow equilibration, and then the pH should be tested. During the equilibration period, visual acuities can be checked and a quick slit-lamp examination can be performed to assess the ocular surface and anterior segment structures. Irrigation should then be continued until a neutral pH of 7.0 is reached.

Once the pH has been normalized, re-examination at the slit lamp should be performed, and cotton-tipped applicators or jeweler forceps should be used to remove the cement debris from the ocular surface. Special care should be taken to check in the inferior fornices and under the upper eyelid in the superior fornices (Figure 43-1). Double eversion of the upper eyelids must be performed to ensure that there is no debris in the upper fornices. It is imperative to ensure that no debris remains as any leftover debris will continue to serve as a reservoir of alkali in the form of lime, which will continue to cause damage. Any areas of frank necrosis of the ocular surface should also be noted and necrotic material should be debrided to remove any residual caustic material and to promote better epithelialization. Once all of the debris and necrosis is removed, irrigation with a few more liters of normal saline should be performed to wash out any residual alkali. Once the pH is confirmed to be normalized, irrigation can be stopped and the eyes should be re-examined once again. The epithelial defects on both the corneas and the conjunctivae should be noted (Figure 43-2) and the intraocular pressures should be checked because alkali burns can frequently cause raised intraocular pressures. The presence of intraocular inflammation should be noted and a special assessment of the limbus should be undertaken to grade the damage based on the Roper-Hall modification of the Hughes classification.[1]

Early Medical Management

Crucial to outcome of the injury now rests with the initial medical management. Contrary to the conservative practices that are frequently employed, the use of an intensive regimen of corticosteroid eye drops is essential to a favorable outcome, and in the fact, the benefit of corticosteroid-induced reduction in inflammation from prolonged use of corticosteroids is not associated with significant corneal stromal melting.[2] Thus, in this case, I would favor the use of prednisolone acetate 1% drops every 2 hours in both eyes. Along with this, I would cover with a broad-spectrum antibiotic drop such as a fourth-generation fluoroquinolone 4 times daily, and I would add a cycloplegic agent such as scopolamine 0.25% 4 times daily or atropine 1% twice daily (not phenylephrine because of its vasoconstrictive properties). Furthermore, I would consider either oral vitamin C 1 g 4 times daily (don't forget to remind the patient to drink a lot of water) or oral doxycycline 100 mg twice daily (or both) to prevent stromal melting.[3] Sodium citrate 10% drops can also be used for this purpose, but it is difficult to obtain and, in this case, is probably not necessary. If the intraocular pressure is elevated, oral acetazolamide 250 mg 4 times daily or 500 mg twice daily can be used, or a topical beta-blocker should be given. Frequent use of preservative-free artificial tears should be encouraged on an hourly basis and, if necessary, an oral analgesic can be prescribed.

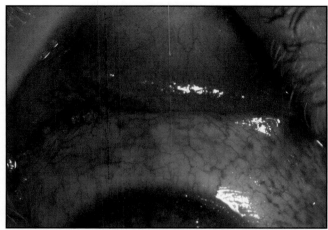

Figure 43-1. Cement particles lodged in the upper fornix of a gentleman who suffered an alkali burn to the eye with cement. Failure to identify and remove these particles will result in a reservoir for continued alkali release onto the ocular surface. (Photo courtesy of Richard L. Abbott, MD.).

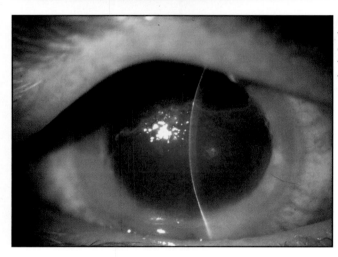

Figure 43-2. Diffuse epithelial disruption of the inferior two-thirds of the cornea after an acute alkali burn to the eye from cement. (Photo courtesy of Richard L. Abbott, MD.).

Amniotic Membrane Grafting for Severe Burns

Unless a Grade IV burn is noted, surgical intervention is typically not necessary at this time. However, in severe burns, amniotic membrane grafting has become a popular modality for treatment.[4] Amniotic membrane possesses nutrients and growth factors that can help suppress inflammation and promote epithelialization. In addition, it can be useful in helping to protect the fragile, damaged ocular surface. Sometimes, the placement of an amniotic membrane is done in conjunction with the placement of a temporary tarsorrhaphy. A new sutureless temporary amniotic membrane patch is also available commercially, and this may prove to be an efficient and efficacious treatment modality during the acute phase of ocular chemical burns.[4]

Ongoing Medical Management

During the first week, medical therapy should be continued and the patient should be seen daily until the epithelium (cornea and conjunctiva) is healed. It is common to

Figure 43-3. Symblepharon formation in the lower fornix several weeks after an alkali burn to the eye with cement. (Photo courtesy of Richard L. Abbott, MD.).

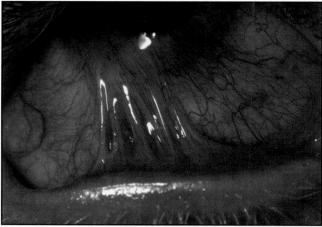

overlook conjunctival defects, which could end up melting and necrosing. Any new areas of necrosis should be treated with debridement, and topical collagenase inhibitors such as acetylcysteine 10% can be used 4 times daily. If perforation is a threat, then a corneal or scleral patch graft (depending on the location of the necrosis) may be warranted. During this time, the intraocular pressure should be monitored and treated, and any conjunctival adhesions in the fornices (Figure 43-3) that are seen can be lysed with a cotton-tipped applicator.

After the first week, the topical corticosteroid drops should be tapered to 4 times daily and, if the epithelium is not healed, consideration should be made to intervene with a bandage contact lens. Aggressive lubrication should also be continued. Alternatively, pressure patching with an antibiotic/corticosteroid combination ointment in the eye is an option. If this is unsuccessful, an amniotic membrane graft with or without a temporary tarsorrhaphy may be warranted at this time. Ultimately, chronic dry eyes and limbal stem cell deficiency can be sequelae of chemical burns that may require long-term or even life-long care. However, that being said, aggressive and prompt initial management of such cases will give the patient the best chance for a more favorable outcome.

References

1. Roper-Hall MJ. Thermal and chemical burns. *Trans Ophthalmol Soc UK*. 1965;85:631-653.
2. Brodovsky SC, McCarty CA, Snibson G, et al. Management of alkali burns. An 11-year retrospective review. *Ophthalmology*. 2000;107(10):1829-1835.
3. Wagoner MD. Chemical injuries of the eye: current concepts in pathophysiology and therapy. *Surv Ophthalmol*. 1997;41(4):275-313.
4. Kheirkhah A, Johnson DA, Paranjpe DR, Raju VK, Casas V, Tseng SC. Temporary sutureless amniotic membrane patch for acute alkaline burns. *Arch Ophthalmol*. 2008;126(8):1059-1066.

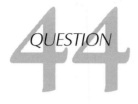

A TIRE BLEW UP IN FRONT OF MY PATIENT'S FACE. HE COMPLAINS OF EYE IRRITATION. THE EXAM SHOWS MULTIPLE TINY FOREIGN BODIES 100 TO 200 µM IN DIAMETER EMBEDDED IN THE CONJUNCTIVA AND CORNEA. DOES HE NEED SURGERY?

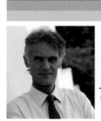

Jose L. Güell, MD
(co-authored with Merce Morral, MD)

Corneal and conjunctival foreign bodies (FB) are one of the most frequent ophthalmic emergencies. Similar to other traumatic injuries, FBs occur most frequently in males younger than 40 years old in their occupational environment and war settings.[1] Materials include metal, glass, wood, plastic, and sand, among others. References on multiple FBs include severe ocular trauma, including ocular perforation and intraocular FBs.[2] Surprisingly, there are no reports of superficial multiple FBs in the peer-reviewed literature.

Clinical Evaluation

After any ocular trauma, visual acuity assessment followed by a complete ophthalmologic evaluation is essential to establish the severity of the damage and visual prognosis. Topical anesthesia (eg, 1 to 2 drops of proparacaine 0.5%) usually facilitates initial exploration. Generally, superficial corneal FBs are much more common than deeply embedded corneal FBs. If the FB is metallic and more than 24 hours have passed from the initial trauma, a rust ring and a ring infiltrate surrounding the object is often seen (Figure 44-1).

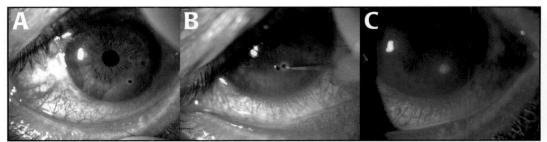

Figure 44-1. Metallic corneal foreign body. A rust ring and a ring infiltrate surrounding the object are seen (A). The rust ring that remains in the cornea after removal of a metallic FB requires removal with a drill or the tip of a needle (B). An epithelial defect remains after removal (C). (Photo courtesy of S. Ortiz, MD.)

It is easier to grasp the metallic superficial FB at this stage than earlier. FBs may cause a small sterile inflammatory reaction around the foreign object. However, if a large infiltrate or significant anterior chamber reaction are present, infectious keratitis is suspected and corneal scraping for smears and cultures should be taken.

Upon examination, this patient case shows multiple tiny FBs at the surface of and embedded within the cornea and conjunctiva. First of all, it is important to ensure that no FB has perforated the cornea and penetrated into the eye. Use the Seidel test to look for corneal or corneoscleral penetration when it is not obvious. An intraocular foreign body (IOFB) that penetrates into the anterior chamber of the eye or into the globe itself is likely to cause significant morbidity that may significantly affect ocular and visual function. The imaging technique of choice when an IOFB is suspected is orbital CT scan (1-mm axial and coronal cuts). Magnetic resonance imaging may also be useful, but it is contraindicated if a metal FB is suspected. B-scan ultrasound and ultrasound biomicroscopy (UBM) may also be useful.[3] Anterior segment optical coherence tomography may also be helpful to evaluate anterior chamber structures in the presence of corneal opacities. These studies should be complemented by a full-dilated examination of the fundus.

Management: Extraction of Foreign Bodies

In the absence of corneal perforation, all superficial and embedded corneal FBs that have not yet epithelialized should be removed as soon as possible to avoid complications such as infectious keratitis or secondary tissue necrosis. When a corneal FB encroaches on the visual axis, patients must be informed of the potential loss of visual acuity due to unavoidable scarring, secondary corneal opacity, and/or irregular astigmatism (Figure 44-2).

Corneal and Conjunctival Foreign Bodies

Under topical anesthesia, a direct stream of sterile irrigating solution may be sufficient to dislodge some small FBs. In the case of FBs on the conjunctival fornix and caruncular area, use a microsponge to eliminate them. If still necessary, a complete ocular surface cleaning should be done with as much irrigating solution as possible, including the conjunctival fornices.

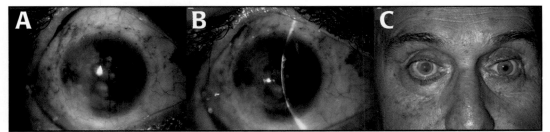

Figure 44-2. Multiple foreign bodies. Multiple foreign bodies on the cornea and conjunctiva after a car battery blew up in front of the face of a patient. The patient did not require any intraocular or corneal surgery, as he presented with best-corrected visual acuity of 20/40 and no ocular inflammation was noticed (A, B). Multiple foreign bodies in both eyes and the face of another patient. His right eye presents BSCVA of counting fingers after vitreoretinal surgery and penetrating keratoplasty. He lost his left eye due to the severe ocular injury (C).

If this is not successful in the cornea, one can use a flexible-loop foreign body spud or 25-gauge needle placed onto a syringe (1 to 3 mL) to remove objects under slit-lamp examination. Some clinicians like to bend the needle at a slight angle. Cotton-tipped applicators or microsponges are less appropriate to eliminate FBs on the cornea because the large surface area of cotton that touches the cornea may potentially create a larger epithelial defect. Rust rings that remain in the cornea after removal of a metallic FB may require removal with a drill. Finally, lids need to be everted to look for additional FBs. After the removal of corneal FBs, check for a negative Seidel sign (especially after using a sharp instrument) to confirm that no iatrogenic penetration of the cornea occurred during the procedure.

FBs embedded in the corneal stroma that have epithelialized and become buried in the cornea may be left in place and observed as long as they are small and inert. However, FBs suspected to have penetrated into the anterior chamber, organic FBs (eg, plants) in any location, or metallic particles should be removed as soon as possible.[4] Although this is an infrequent phenomenon, metallic FBs left in the eye may cause irreversible ocular damage at all levels, which is known as ocular siderosis.[5] FBs that present any potential for intraocular penetration should be removed in the operating room within 24 hours of initial examination. If the FB is located in deep stroma, it is sometimes easier and less destructive to the stroma to push the FB into the anterior chamber and remove it through a peripheral paracentesis under viscoelastic protection and using a vitreoretinal forceps.

Medical Treatment, Follow-Up, and Patient Counseling

After removal, topical broad-spectrum antibiotic drops or ointment and a topical cycloplegic should be prescribed until the epithelial defect heals to prevent infection. As long as infection has been ruled out and antibiotics have been instilled for at least 24 hours, topical steroids should be used if inflammatory signs are present. However, steroids should be used cautiously as they increase the likelihood of infection and slow healing.

Corneal erosions may be associated with moderate to severe pain. Thus, oral analgesia may be required. Topical anesthetics prolong epithelial healing and should be avoided for pain relief. Topical cycloplegics (cyclopentolate 1% once or twice daily) may be used in cases of moderate to severe pain. Although nonsteroidal anti-inflammatory drug ophthalmic solutions (eg, ketorolac) have been described to provide significant pain relief and have not been found to slow healing, we do not recommend their use.[6] Without patching, patients note faster healing, less blurred vision, and even less pain. Thus, patching is only recommended to protect abrasions that cover more than 50% of the cornea.[7]

A close follow-up is required until the epithelial defect is well healed and any corneal infiltrates have resolved. Moreover, patient education is essential to prevent further episodes of ocular trauma. Patients need to be advised to wear safety goggles in any situation that has a high risk of particles or objects flying into the eyes. In those cases with multiple metallic FBs, a long-term follow-up is recommended to allow early diagnosis of late inflammation and siderosis.

As far as visual prognosis is concerned, superficial foreign bodies that are removed soon after the injury usually leave no permanent sequelae. However, corneal scarring or infection may occur and affect visual acuity, especially if they are located at the central or paracentral corneal area. Depending on the depth of the residual stromal scar, phototherapeutic keratectomy (PTK) or deep anterior lamellar keratoplasty may be required to restore visual function. In the case of IOFB and ocular perforation, visual prognosis depends on the acute and late damage to intraocular structures and the appearance of postoperative complications, such as retinal detachment or endophthalmitis.

References

1. Gumus K, Karakucuk S, Mirza E. Corneal injury from a metallic foreign body: an occupational hazard. *Eye Contact Lens*. 2007;33(5):259-260.
2. Thach AB, Ward TP, Dick JS 2nd, et al. Intraocular foreign body injuries during Operation Iraqi Freedom. *Ophthalmology*. 2005;112(10):1829-1833.
3. Deramo VA, Shah GK, Baumal CR, et al. Ultrasound biomicroscopy as a tool for detecting and localizing occult foreign bodies after ocular trauma. *Ophthalmology*. 1999;106(2):301-305.
4. Chen WL, Tseng CH, Wang IJ, Hu FR. Removal of semitranslucent cactus spines embedded in deep cornea with the aid of a fiberoptic illuminator. *Am J Ophthalmol*. 2002;134(5):769-771.
5. Talamo JH, Topping TM, Maumenee AE, Green WR. Ultrastructural studies of cornea, iris and lens in a case of siderosis bulbi. *Ophthalmology*. 1985;92(12):1675-1680.
6. Guidera AC, Luchs JI, Udell IJ. Keratitis, ulceration, and perforation associated with topical nonsteroidal anti-inflammatory drugs. *Ophthalmology*. 2001;108(5):936-944.
7. Turner A, Rabiu M. Patching for corneal abrasion. *Cochrane Database Syst Rev*. 2006;(2):CD004764.

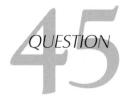
A PATIENT WITH A CHEMICAL BURN IN THE RIGHT EYE 6 MONTHS AGO COMPLAINS OF BLURRY VISION AND PHOTOPHOBIA. HE HAS AN AREA OF CORNEAL NEOVASCULARIZATION AND CONJUNCTIVALIZATION EXTENDING 4 MM FROM THE LIMBUS. DOES HE NEED LIMBAL STEM CELL TRANSPLANTATION?

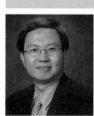

Scheffer C. G. Tseng, MD, PhD
(co-authored with Hosam Sheha, MD, PhD)

The integrity of the corneal epithelium is ultimately dictated by its stem cells, which are located at the limbus. Therefore, a significant loss of limbal stem cells and/or their supporting limbal stroma will lead to one major type of ocular surface failure, termed *limbal stem cell deficiency* (LSCD). Patients inflicted with LSCD will frequently manifest annoying photophobia and a significant loss of vision. Although LSCD is a common outcome, not all eyes that have a past history of chemical burn exhibit LSCD. The mere presence of poor epithelial integrity (irregular surface, recurrent erosion, or persistent defect), superficial vascularization, and pannus is not sufficient for one to make the diagnosis of LSCD in chemically burned corneas. This is because these clinical signs can also be induced by other types of ocular surface failure resulting from chemical burns such as dry eye, exposure, neurotrophic state, and blink-related microtrauma from lids and lashes. The hallmark of LSCD lies in "conjunctivalization" (ie, invasion of conjunctival epithelium onto the cornea), which clinically can be suggested by "late fluorescein staining," but definitely confirmed by impression cytology.[1] A clear diagnosis of LSCD in a chemically burned eye is critical for the patient to be subjected to appropriate medical and surgical management.

What Are the Treatment Options?

Once the diagnosis of LSCD is confirmed, clinical management depends on the presence of symptoms and the extent of LSCD. If the eye with LSCD is free of any symptom and still has good central vision because the majority of the central corneal epithelium remains intact, management is directed to preserving the integrity of the remaining corneal epithelium. Hence, it is important to use non-preserved artificial tears for lubrication and to consider extended wear of a high-DK bandage contact lens or scleral lens. The latter measure is particularly useful if the eye also presents with superficial punctate keratopathy, dry eye, or infrequent blinking. Because chemical burn may also damage other parts of the ocular surface, surgical treatments directed toward restoring the ocular surface integrity may ameliorate further attrition of the central corneal epithelium. These methods include punctal occlusion for dry eye, tarsorrhaphy for exposure, and plastic surgeries for lid/lash abnormalities. One should resist the temptation to perform epithelial debridement or superficial keratectomy in an attempt to smooth the remaining corneal epithelium because such a procedure will invariably hasten deterioration. Periodic monitoring of the progression is mandatory to ensure the aforementioned vigilant preservation of the remaining central corneal epithelium. Any notable progression will prompt one to search for new causes threatening the ocular surface integrity. In the event that LSCD diagnosis is established, its progression can be judged clinically by the extent of vascularization or late fluorescein staining.

If the eye has annoying photophobia (sometimes to the extent of affecting the vision of the uninvolved fellow eye due to blepharospasm) and/or a notable loss of vision because the central corneal epithelium is threatened or lost, clinical management resorts to restoration of limbal stem cells. If the extent of LSCD is partial (not involving the entire limbus), one novel way of achieving this goal is to transplant cryopreserved amniotic membrane (AmnioGraft, Bio-Tissue, Inc, Miami, FL). This surgical procedure, initially reported in 2001, has recently transitioned to a "sutureless" method facilitated by the use of fibrin glue for partial LSCD.[2] The surgical procedure involves the removal of conjunctivalized pannus from the corneal surface and conjunctival recession via relaxing incision toward the fornix (Figure 45-1), intraoperative application of mitomycin C in the fornix, attachment of AmnioGraft to the denuded perilimbal sclera and corneal surface using fibrin glue (Figure 45-2), and insertion of ProKera (Bio-Tissue, Inc), which is a symblepharon ring fastened with AmnioGraft as a biological bandage (Figure 45-3) (visit www.osref.org for more details and a surgical video). As reported in partial LSCD,[2] the above surgical procedure is capable of restoring the corneal surface by expanding limbal stem cells in the limbal deficient area. For nearly total LSCD, a 2-stage approach of the above surgical procedures is advisable.

If the eye has total LSCD, corneal surface reconstruction relies on transplantation of autologous limbal stem cells from the fellow eye using conjunctival limbal autograft. In this scenario, amniotic membrane transplantation can also be performed to reduce the size of the conjunctival limbal autograft[3] and to restore the limbal integrity in the donor eye.[4] Following the removal of the entire conjunctivalized pannus from the limbal deficient eye, AmnioGraft is secured to the denuded corneal and perilimbal scleral surfaces by fibrin glue. One or 2 free conjunctival limbal autografts, each spanning 2 clock hours, are removed from superior or inferior limbal regions, respectively, and the defect of the

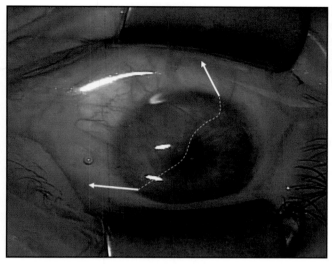

Figure 45-1. In this eye with partial limbal stem cell deficiency, the conjunctivalized pannus is removed by superficial keratectomy and the adjacent conjunctiva is recessed to the fornix (arrows).

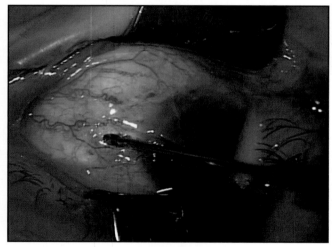

Figure 45-2. The entire denuded corneal and scleral surface is covered by a layer of cryoperserved amniotic membrane with the stromal surface facing down using fibrin glue.

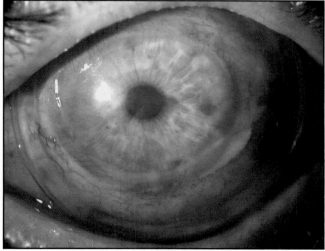

Figure 45-3. ProKera is inserted as a temporary bandage to facilitate healing.

Figure 45-4. In this eye with total limbal stem cell deficiency, conjunctival limbal autograft is secured over AmnioGraft by interrupted 10-0 nylon sutures to the recipient limbal region.

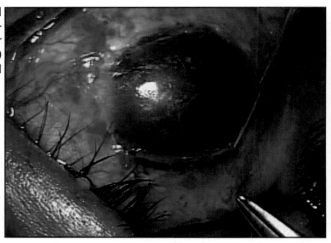

donor site is covered by AmnioGraft using fibrin glue. The conjunctival limbal autograft is then secured over AmnioGraft by interrupted 10-0 nylon sutures to the recipient limbal region (Figure 45-4). Finally, a ProKera is placed on the eye. This surgical procedure is capable of restoring the corneal surface of total LSCD by expanding limbal stem cells in the limbal deficient area.

References

1. Puangsricharern V, Tseng SC. Cytologic evidence of corneal diseases with limbal stem cell deficiency. *Ophthalmology.* 1995;102(10):1476-1485.
2. Kheirkhah A, Casas V, Raju VK, Tseng SC. Sutureless amniotic membrane transplantation for partial limbal stem cell deficiency. *Am J Ophthalmol.* 2008;145(5):787-794.
3. Kheirkhah A, Raju VK, Tseng SC. Minimal conjunctival limbal autograft for total limbal stem cell deficiency. *Cornea.* 2008;27(6):730-733.
4. Meallet MA, Espana EM, Grueterich M, Ti S-E, Goto E, Tseng SCG. Amniotic membrane transplantation for recipient and donor eyes undergoing conjunctival limbal autograft for total limbal stem cell deficiency. *Ophthalmology.* 2003;110:1585-1592.

SECTION VI

POSTOPERATIVE

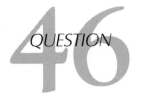

QUESTION 46

WHAT SHOULD I CONSIDER FOR A PATIENT WITH A CORNEAL TRANSPLANT WHO PRESENTS WITH A RED EYE AND PHOTOPHOBIA?

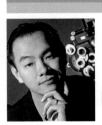

David S. Chu, MD

The differential diagnosis of red eyes with photophobia spans a broad range of pathophysiology; however, a prior history of penetrating keratoplasty makes certain etiologies more likely. These include corneal graft rejection, bullous keratopathy, microbial keratitis, and herpetic keratitis. Other conditions, such as viral keratoconjunctivitis, blepharitis, and allergic conjunctivitis, are generally common conditions but are less frequent in corneal graft recipients. Nevertheless, correct diagnosis is essential as the treatment differs. Furthermore, proactive treatment of inflammatory conditions other than corneal rejection may prevent inciting immunological rejection in the graft.

Graft Rejection

The eye is an immunologically privileged site where the body can actively develop antigenic tolerance. Therefore, cornea transplants have a high success rate without routine systemic immunosuppressants. Corneal graft rejection probability rises with increased corneal neovascularization.[1] Presence of ocular inflammation, glaucoma, limbus dysfunction, trauma, and history of trauma are associated with corneal graft rejection.[2]

Along with redness and photophobia, corneal graft rejection can present with decreased vision, pain, and tearing. Clinical signs include Khoudadoust line (endothelial rejection line), epithelial rejection line, corneal edema, corneal haze, keratic precipitates, corneal infiltrates, corneal neovascularization, and anterior chamber cellular reaction (Figure 46-1).

215

Figure 46-1. Acute corneal graft rejection. A red eye with Khodadoust line, corneal edema, and corneal neovascularization invading into the graft.

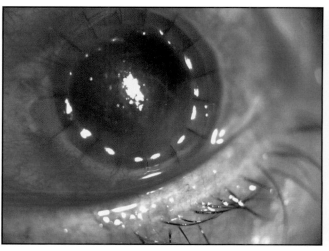

Acute graft rejection episodes of cornea are common, but they are usually controllable with medical therapy. Cases of suspected graft rejection confirmed by examination require immediate anti-inflammatory treatment. I recommend topical prednisolone acetate 1% every 2 hours while awake with dosage modulation for degree of inflammation. Difluprednate 0.05% has recently become available in the United States. Though data are limited, difluprednate may be more potent than prednisolone acetate in controlling anterior segment inflammation and may be useful in treating graft rejection. With both medications, intraocular pressure must be carefully monitored and treated. Loteprednol 0.5% has less likelihood of inducing steroid response; however, in my practice, it's a weaker topical steroid compared with prednisolone acetate and is used only when intraocular pressure control is difficult. In severe acute rejection episodes, oral steroids and regional injections should be considered.

Ophthalmologists do not routinely use systemic solid organ transplant rejection medications, such as mycophenylate mofetil, cyclosporine A, tacrolimus, or daclizumab; however, when benefits outweigh potential risks, they should be considered. Preliminary data suggest topical and regional bevacizumab also show promise in reduction of corneal neovascularization and may be beneficial adjuncts in corneal graft rejection prevention and treatment.[3] Following resolution of the acute episode, the patient may require chronic low-dose topical steroids.

Bullous Keratopathy

Repeated corneal graft rejection can cause endothelial failure and associated bullous keratopathy. In addition to red eyes and photophobia, patients may report tearing and pain. Usually, the edema involves the entire graft (both stromal and epithelial edema). When bullae rupture, the symptoms can worsen, and microbial keratitis may develop.

Placement of a bandage contact lens can swiftly relieve patients' symptoms. However, this is a short-term solution, and patients should be maintained on prophylactic topical antibiotics while using the lens. In eyes without visual prognosis, consider conjunctival flap or amniotic membrane graft placed via "in-lay" technique. AMG can also be a temporary solution if corneal tissue is unavailable or the patient wishes to defer another corneal transplantation. Definitive treatments for these patients are penetrating keratoplasty or endothelial keratoplasty.

Microbial Keratitis and Herpetic Keratitis

Eyes with corneal grafts are at increased risk of developing microbial keratitis from altered ocular surfaces, altered corneal sensation, and presence of corneal sutures (Figure 46-2). Remove loose corneal sutures to prevent microbial keratitis. In patients with bullous keratopathy from failing or failed grafts, there is increased risk for microbial keratitis. Bandage contact lenses placed to treat bullous keratopathy also increase the risk of microbial keratitis.

History of herpetic keratitis is one of the more common reasons for corneal transplant in the United States. Unfortunately, recurrence of herpetic keratitis is common in corneal grafts.

Microbial keratitis and herpetic keratitis may present atypically in patients with corneal grafts; however, prompt diagnosis and treatment of these etiologies is necessary as inflammation from these conditions can frequently lead to vision-altering corneal scars and/or potentially inciting immunological graft rejection.

Other Causes of Red Eyes

Viral keratoconjunctivitis, blepharoconjunctivitis, and allergic conjunctivitis are all common causes of red eye. Their frequently overlapping symptoms and clinical findings with corneal graft rejection sometimes hinders establishment of proper diagnoses. Alteration of the eye and ocular surfaces in corneal graft patients can result in more complex presentations with amplified diagnostic challenges. All of these conditions have prominent itching and burning sensations as well as redness and photophobia in common. Mucoid or watery discharge, usually absent in corneal graft rejection, can be seen.

Clinically, patients present with conjunctivitis, frequently with significant papillary or follicular reactions not seen in corneal graft rejection. However, these conditions can also share some findings with corneal graft rejection. Subepithelial infiltrates, though uncommon, have been reported in corneal graft rejection.[4] Corneal neovascularization is occasionally seen in severe chronic cases of blepharoconjunctivitis and atopic keratoconjunctivitis. Extrapolating from data on increased incidence of corneal graft rejection in eyes with concurrent ocular inflammatory diseases, these conditions must be treated proactively when identified in patients with previous corneal grafts.

Summary

When evaluating and treating red eyes in patients with a history of corneal transplantation, physicians must carefully differentiate the causes of red eyes, as some of the signs and symptoms overlap in the list of differentials. Graft rejections should be treated aggressively, as should non-rejection inflammatory conditions, as they may incite graft rejection episodes.

Figure 46-2. Bacterial keratitis in a corneal graft with loose sutures.

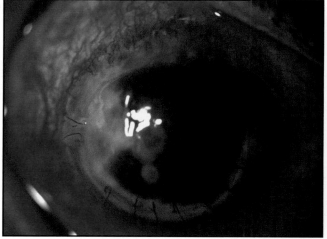

References

1. Khoudadoust AA, Karnema Y. Corneal grafts in the second eye. *Cornea.* 1984;3(1):17-20.
2. Maguire MG, Stark WJ, Gottsch JD, et al. Risk factors for corneal graft failure and rejection in the collaborative corneal transplantation studies. Collaborative Corneal Transplantation Studies Research Group. *Ophthalmology.* 1994;101(9):1536-1547.
3. Doctor PP, Bhat PV, Foster CS. Subconjunctival bevacizumab for corneal neovascularization. *Cornea.* 2008;27(9):992-995.
4. Krachmer JH, Alldredge OC. Subepithelial infiltrates: a probable sign of corneal graft rejection. *Arch Ophthalmol.* 1978;96(12):2234-2237.

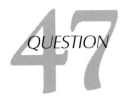

How Should I Manage an Intraocular Pressure Spike of 43 mm Hg in a Descemet's Stripping Endothelial Keratoplasty Patient Who Is Taking One Drop of Pred Forte 1% Daily?

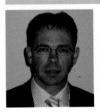

Rudy M. M. A. Nuijts, MD, PhD
(co-authored with Muriel Doors, MD;
Carroll A. Webers, MD, PhD; and Nienke Visser, MD)

Elevated intraocular pressure after corneal transplantation is a common problem due to the long-term use of steroid drops to prevent graft rejection. High steroid responses (IOP >21 mm Hg) may occur in more than 15% of transplant patients.

IOP Measurement After DSEK

The interpretation of the IOP in transplants with an increased corneal thickness may be challenging. It has been postulated that a 10% change in central corneal thickness will result in a 3.4 mm Hg change of IOP. After Descemet's stripping endothelial keratoplasty (DSEK), the corneal thickness may increase to around 690 μm.[1] Goldmann tonometer is calibrated for a corneal thickness of 520 μm and, therefore, Goldmann tonometry is less accurate in corneas with a thickness out of the normal range. Nomograms to correct for the falsely increased IOP in thick corneas are not commonly used because their accuracy is questionable. It has been suggested that dynamic contour tonometry (DCT; PASCAL, Swiss Microtechnology, Zurich, Switzerland) measures IOP independent from curvature and corneal thickness. In a recent study comparing IOP after DSEK with 3 measurement techniques (Goldmann tonometry, DCT, and pneumatonometry), it was shown that Goldmann tonometry measured lower IOP levels (4 mm Hg lower on average) as compared to DCT and pneumatonometry.[2] In addition, no correlation was found between IOP and corneal thickness. Because the graft is not attached to the limbus, these findings suggest that the DSEK part of the cornea does not contribute to the biomechanical effects on IOP measurement (Figure 47-1). It is also possible that the viscous properties of the DSEK cornea have changed because of the graft or the resolution of previous corneal edema, which could be responsible for the lower IOP measured by Goldmann tonometry.

IOP-Lowering Eye Drops

Most likely, a patient with intraocular pressure elevation after DSEK is a steroid responder, and my preferred treatment would be a topical non-selective beta-adrenergic blocker, such as timolol. My second choice would be an adrenergic agonist. However, other causes of late postoperative IOP elevations, including damage to the trabecular meshwork, persistent inflammation, or pre-existing glaucoma, have to be considered.

General principles of medical glaucoma treatment can be summarized as follows.[3] Initial therapy constitutes of monotherapy with a first-choice group (in alphabetical order) of α_2-adrenergic agonists, beta blockers, topical carbonic anhydrase inhibitors, and prostaglandin analogs. If the drug is effective and there are no side effects, the regimen will be continued. Often, an IOP decrease of at least 20% from baseline is defined as an effective initial treatment. If the first-choice drug is not effective or if side effects occur, then therapy is switched within the first-choice group. Even if the drug is effective but the target IOP is not reached, a switch between monotherapies is an option. However, if the first drug has decreased IOP sufficiently but the target IOP is not reached, combining drugs from the first-choice group is the next step. Combining 3 drugs, preferably 2 in a fixed form, is considered maximum medical therapy. Adding another drug to a combination of 3 drugs does not result in significant additional IOP lowering. Non-selective adrenergic agents, parasymphaticomimetics, and systemic carbonic anhydrase inhibitors are considered a second-choice group. Treatment of high IOP with carbonic anhydrase inhibitors may have an adverse effect on corneal endothelial cells by attenuating the bicarbonate efflux and subsequent loss of stroma dehydration. Dorzolamide has been reported to lead to increased corneal thickness, but the effect on corneal cell morphology and corneal cell density is unknown. However, carbonic anhydrase inhibitor therapy may have a stronger effect on corneal thickness in patients with pre-existing corneal endothelium problems (such as those due to Fuchs' endothelial dystrophy or following penetrating keratoplasty), which has also been suggested in the literature.[4,5] Even though the effect of carbonic anhydrase inhibitors on corneal endothelium is not fully elucidated, I suggest to be careful with dorzolamide in patients with a compromised corneal endothelium. Concomitant oral therapy might even enhance the effects of topical carbonic anhydrase on corneal endothelium.

Minimizing the Likelihood of Steroid Responses

To prevent steroid responses in the future, a topical steroid with the least chance to increase IOP should be chosen. The ability of topical steroids to induce IOP elevation

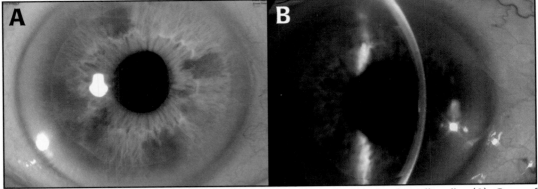

Figure 47-1. Case of DSEK showing a clear, nicely centered posterior lamellar disc (A). Case of DSEK showing the posterior lamellar disc that is not attached to the limbus and therefore has no biomechanical effect on measuring IOP (B).

depends on the dosage, treatment duration, drug formulation (hydrophilic phosphate form or lipophilic alcohol or acetate form), and the anti-inflammatory potency of the steroid. Dexamethasone and prednisolone are highly potent steroids and cause steroid responses more often than less potent steroids. Fluorometholone and rimexolone are effective in controlling ocular inflammation but lead to substantially less IOP elevation. This is possibly due to a local steroid metabolism in the cornea and subsequent reduced penetration into the aqueous humor. Consequently, because of the long-term steroid treatment to prevent graft rejection in DSEK patients, fluormetholone or rimexolone should be preferred over prednisolone and dexamethasone. In addition, tapering the dose of steroids and/or using a lower steroid concentration could be used to reduce IOP further. In case-elevated IOP persists despite lowering the corticosteroid dose and initiating anti-glaucomatous drugs, a switch to systemic immunosuppressive drugs (eg, cyclosporine, mycophenolate mofetil, etc) could be considered in patients with high risk for immune graft rejection.

References

1. Price MO, Price FW Jr. Descemet's stripping with endothelial keratoplasty: comparative outcomes with micro-keratome-dissected and manually dissected donor tissue. *Ophthalmology.* 2006;113(11):1936-1942.
2. Vajaranant TS, Price MO, Price FW, Wilensky JT, Edward DP. Intraocular pressure measurements following Descemet stripping endothelial keratoplasty. *Am J Ophthalmol.* 2008;145(5):780-786.
3. Webers CA, Beckers HJ, Nuijts RM, Schouten JS. Pharmacological management of primary open-angle glaucoma: second-line options and beyond. *Drugs Aging.* 2008;25(9):729-759.
4. Konowal A, Morrison JC, Brown SV, et al. Irreversible corneal decompensation in patients treated with topical dorzolamide. *Am J Ophthalmol.* 1999;127(4):403-406.
5. Wirtitsch MG, Findl O, Heinzl H, Drexler W. Effect of dorzolamide hydrochloride on central corneal thickness in humans with cornea guttata. *Arch Ophthalmol.* 2007;125(10):1345-1350.

I Was Asked to Assume Follow-Up of a Patient 5 Months After Penetrating Keratoplasty for HSV-Related Scar. How Should I Manage This Patient?

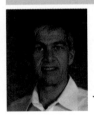

Joseph Tauber, MD

With continued advancement in surgical techniques, selective corneal transplantation is quickly becoming the standard of care in the surgical rehabilitation of corneal disease. Aside from the technical challenges of LK, PK, DSEK, DMEK, and DALK, postoperative decision making requires astute clinical judgment, experience, and recognition of warning signs of the myriad potential complications that lay ahead after the patch is removed on postop day 1. In my residency, the need to combine a "medical approach" with surgical treatment was summarized for me in 2 simple aphorisms: "Surgery is nothing more than cutting and stitching" and "you can teach a monkey *how* to operate, but not *when* to operate." The case described above presents many issues for consideration, highlighting the need to "think" after we "cut."

What Can Be Done to Minimize the Risk of Immunologic Graft Rejection?

For the patient, immune rejection of the graft is the most feared postoperative complication. It has long been reported that the risk of graft rejection is highest and remains constant during the first 2 to 3 years after keratoplasty,[1] but may occur as long as 31 years after surgery.[2] I have personally seen rejection occur 26 years after PK. Of course, the risk of rejection is the key issue guiding decisions to maintain prophylactic anti-rejection therapy over time. Topical corticosteroids are the mainstay of prophylaxis of immune rejection, but cyclosporine and other immunomodulators may be used. Corticosteroids are highly effective as treatment of active rejection, with 50% to 90% reversal of findings of rejection in reports of low-risk populations. The primary complications limiting perpetual corticosteroid therapy are elevation of intraocular pressure and cataract. No published study has compared schedules of corticosteroid taper after grafting, leaving great variability in treatment regimens between physicians. A standardized taper protocol was devised and used in the multicenter Collaborative Corneal Transplantation Study[3] as well as in several more recent studies, and is the best available guide to an agreed upon standard schedule. Superstition often overrides scientific data, with many clinicians choosing to maintain their PK patients on low-dose corticosteroids for life at doses of once or twice weekly. Some experts recommend tapering off corticosteroids within 6 months of grafting, especially in low-risk, phakic patients, but indefinite low-dose treatment in high-risk patients (eg, vascularization or prior rejection).[4] I have found minimal complications to indefinite treatment with loteprednol or fluorometholone every 2 to 3 days, and I typically maintain almost all of my PK patients on some corticosteroid for life. I do not maintain lifelong corticosteroid treatment in keratoconic or non-inflammatory pediatric cases unless there are exceptional high-risk features.

When and How Should Sutures Be Removed?

The decision to remove sutures following PK must balance the tectonic support that sutures provide against the infectious risks of suture-related abscess, microbial keratitis, and endophthalmitis. Spontaneous wound dehiscence has been reported even 2 years after removal of corneal sutures, and traumatic wound rupture is a dreaded lifelong risk following PK. Refractive changes occur after suture removal, even years following surgery, complicating the decision to remove sutures in all patients even if the refractive result is good. Clinicians must consider patient age as wound healing is much slower in the elderly. Any suture that is vascularized or loose must be removed. In patients under age 50, my practice is to remove all sutures by 12 to 18 months following surgery. In older patients, I leave sutures in place unless removal is indicated for refractive modification, vascularization, or laxity. Suture removal is advisable in patients not compliant with follow-up visits who are more likely to present with broken and infected sutures. The advent of femtosecond laser-assisted keratoplasty may increase the tectonic stability of the keratoplasty wound and permit earlier removal of sutures, but this will require future studies.

How Should the Patient Be Monitored for an Immunologic Rejection Reaction?

Establishing a schedule for routine follow-up and monitoring for rejection is important. My usual follow-up schedule is day 1, week 1, month 1, every 4 to 6 weeks for the first 6 months, every 2 to 3 months through the first year, and then every 4 to 6 months thereafter. Many factors impact the timing of these visits, including the refractive status, degree of inflammation, epithelial integrity, IOP, and patient reliability and compliance. Routine postoperative visits should include corneal pachymetry at every visit, as a 10% increase in corneal thickness may be an early warning of graft complications, even without endothelial precipitates or clinically evident edema.[5]

How Can the Risk of Herpetic Keratitis Recurrence Be Minimized?

Patients with a history of herpetic keratitis are at increased risk for recurrence following keratoplasty. Long-term prophylactic therapy with oral antiviral agents is recommended in at-risk patients for at least 1 year following keratoplasty[6-9] to reduce the risks of both graft rejection and HSV recurrence. No report has demonstrated superiority of a particular antiviral drug, and compliance and cost considerations must be balanced in individual patients. I typically treat with generic acyclovir 400 mg 3 times a day for 6 months, and then twice daily for the following 6 months. Despite literature to support the effectiveness of 200 mg twice daily in suppression of genital HSV, I believe higher doses are needed after PK. I generally maintain treatment for 12 months following any herpetic flare-up in my keratoplasty patients. Side effects or drug intolerance is rare, but I have the impression that strains of resistant HSV are more prevalent over the past decade, with breakthrough recurrences seen despite treatment with each of the 3 available oral prophylactic agents.

Summary

The surgical procedure of penetrating keratoplasty is only the beginning of a long-term relationship between the surgeon and the patient. Sustained diligence is necessary to optimize visual outcomes.

References

1. Boisjoly HM, Roy R, Bernard PM, Dubé I, Laughrea PA, Bazin R. Association between corneal allograft reactions and HLA compatibility. *Ophthalmology*. 1990;97(12):1689-1698.
2. Chandler JW. Immunologic considerations in corneal transplantation. In Kaufman HE, Barron BA, McDonald MB, Waltman SR, eds. *The Cornea*. New York, NY: Churchill Livingstone; 1988.
3. The Collaborative Corneal Transplantation Studies Research Group. Design and methods of The Collaborative Corneal Transplantation Studies. *Cornea*. 1993;12(2):93-103.
4. Nguyen NX, Seitz B, Martus P, Langenbucher A, Cursiefen C. Long-term topical steroid treatment improves graft survival following normal-risk penetrating keratoplasty. *Am J Ophthalmology*. 2007;144(2):318-319.
5. McDonnell PJ, Enger C, Stark WJ, Stulting RD. Corneal thickness changes after high risk penetrating keratoplasty. Collaborative Corneal Transplantation Study Group. *Arch Ophthalmol*. 1993;111(10):1374-1381.
6. Moyes AL, Sugar A, Musch DC, Barnes RD. Antiviral therapy after penetrating keratoplasty for Herpes Simplex keratitis. *Arch Ophthalmol*. 1994;112(5):601-607.
7. van Rooij J, Rijneveld WJ, Remeijer L, et al. Effect of oral acyclovir after penetrating keratoplasty for herpetic keratitis: a placebo-controlled multicenter trial. *Ophthalmology*. 2003;110(10):1916-1919.

8. Simon AL, Pavan-Langston D. Long-term oral acyclovir therapy. Effect on recurrent infectious herpes simplex keratitis in patients with and without grafts. *Ophthalmology.* 1996;103(9):1399-1404.
9. Barney NP, Foster CS. A prospective randomized trial of oral acyclovir after penetrating keratoplasty for herpes simplex keratitis. *Cornea.* 1994;13(3):232-236.

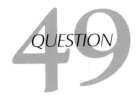

WHAT SHOULD I DO FOR A PATIENT WHO PRESENTS WITH 6-D ASTIGMATISM AFTER UNDERGOING PENETRATING KERATOPLASTY 4 MONTHS AGO?

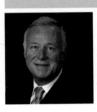

Roger F. Steinert, MD

Consider a contact lens first. A rigid gas-permeable contact lens is always the safest manner to correct both regular and irregular (high-order aberration) astigmatism, whether early or late postoperatively. The following responses assume that an adequate contact lens fitting has been attempted with unacceptable results.

Suture Removal: When and Where?

Because the sutures are in place and the patient is only 4 months after surgery, initial management consists of selective suture removal of any interrupted sutures, followed by adjustment of the tension in the running suture if a running suture is present. The fundamental concept is that the steep hemi-meridian, as evidenced by higher power or steepness on corneal topography, will be improved by reduction in tight sutures in that hemi-meridian (Figure 49-1).

My personal preference is to perform a single running 24 bite 10-0 nylon suture closure on all penetrating keratoplasty (PK) patients where there is no contraindication. Contraindications include vascularization, prior problems with wound healing, or a risk of trauma or pressure on the transplant incision. When a running suture is present, suture-in astigmatism is improved with adjustment of suture tension at the slit lamp with topical anesthesia and a jeweler's forceps. Lax suture tension in the flatter, lower

Figure 49-1. More than 4 D of astigmatism in a postoperative PK patient (A). Reduction to 1.1 D astigmatism by adjusting the tension on the running suture, tightening the lower power areas at lower right and upper left, and moving the lax suture to the steeper, higher power areas at upper right and lower left (B).

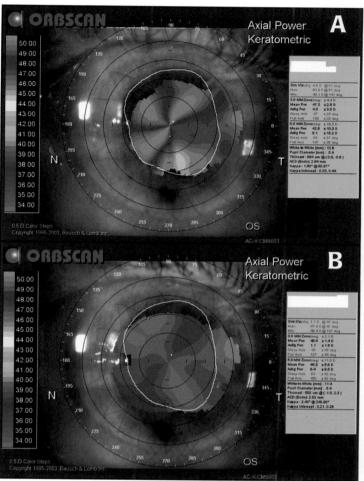

power hemi-meridian is the starting point. The forceps is used to pull on the suture and generate some lax suture material. This excess suture is then moved into the area of the tight/steep cornea. If the suture material in this area is tight, then reducing the tension will improve the astigmatism. A running suture closure for PK has been shown to result in less suture-in astigmatism and more rapid recovery of good visual acuity than a combined interrupted and running suture technique.[1]

Other interventions for reduction of astigmatism usually should wait until full removal of all sutures. Otherwise, the distortion of remaining sutures may result in shifts in any astigmatic correction. The timing of safe full suture removal is a subjective judgment. In general, the appearance of some degree of gray haze at the incision is necessary before one can have any degree of confidence that wound healing has occurred. The older the patient and the more peripheral edema in the cornea, the slower the establishment of wound integrity independent of the sutures. Corneal surgeons have experienced wound separation that requires repair after suture removal 4 or more years after initial surgery in elderly patients who had pseudophakic edema. Conversely, most keratoconus patients younger than 30 years will have good wound integrity 6 to 12 months postoperatively. None of these guidelines are concrete, however.

If a patient has had maximal suture removal and/or release of tension of a running suture in the steep/high power area, yet the hemi-meridian continues to show steepness/excess optical power, there is one intermediate intervention to consider when sutures remain. Under topical anesthesia at the slit lamp, a jeweler's forceps can be used to pry open the anterior aspect of the incision in the steep area. This release of the anterior healed area may allow the tissues to shift so that the donor cornea elevates relative to the recipient rim, reducing the optical power in that zone.

After full suture removal, astigmatism tends to regress toward the mean.[2] Patients with low astigmatism will, on average, have an increase in astigmatism, and patients with high astigmatism will, on average, have improvement. No investigation has conclusively proven a permanent improvement in suture-out astigmatism because of suture manipulations in the earlier postoperative period. This does not mean that suture manipulations are a waste of time. Many PK patients will retain sutures for many years after surgery, and the astigmatism with sutures in place is important for a number of years.

Astigmatic Keratotomy

The easiest and least expensive surgical intervention is astigmatic keratotomy. Because the source of the astigmatism is the graft-host junction, I place these incisions slightly inside the g-h junction. Use of a peripheral incision (limbal relaxing incision) is much less powerful and has the additional disadvantage of creating a shift in the normal part of the cornea. If there is a later re-graft, this distortion will still be present.

Astigmatic keratotomy inside the graft-host junction can be quite powerful because the tissue is under abnormal levels of stress compared to virgin corneas. Therefore, I reduce the amount of the correction by 50% compared to the amount predicted by the formulas for virgin cornea astigmatic keratotomy at that diameter. Even then, overcorrections may occur. An overcorrection should be treated by cleaning the epithelial plug out of the AK incision and suturing the incision closed for several months. Undercorrection is treated by lengthening the original incision or, if the incision is already long, adding a second incision 0.5 mm inside the original AK.

AK incisions are best when the astigmatism is regular (geometrically symmetrical). Conversely, the more asymmetric, the less reliable AK will be (Figure 49-2).

Laser Refractive Surgery

In theory, less symmetrical astigmatism, which means higher-order aberration, should be treated with wavefront-guided (NOT "wavefront-optimized") laser correction. The surgeon must first determine whether the diagnostic wavefront unit can capture the highly aberrated optics and create a treatment plan that has parameters that match the clinical determinations. If so, the patient must understand that the treatment is "off-label" in the United States because the FDA approval of wavefront-guided corrections is for primary treatments, where low-order aberrations (sphere and cylinder) are high and high-order aberrations are low. This is usually not the case for PK optics.

Figure 49-2. Partially asymmetric astigmatism. The hemimeridian at lower right has more power than the upper left, but the bow-tie shape is orthogonal. This could be treated with a larger AK in the lower right than the length of the AK in the upper left or, alternatively, with wavefront-guided corneal ablation. A more symmetrical and lower power residual astigmatism could then be resolved with a toric intraocular lens (IOL) implant.

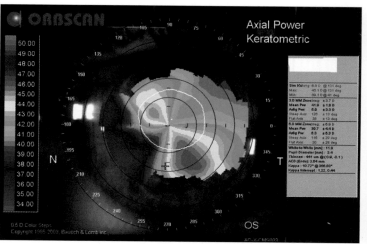

If laser corneal surgery is undertaken, the primary options are either PRK with mitomycin C to reduce haze or LASIK with the femtosecond laser. A microkeratome will usually cut across the PK incision and create astigmatic shifts, as well as risk buttonholes. A femtosecond laser can be programmed to create a flap entirely inside the PK incision.

Any corneal surgery after prior PK increases the potential for immune rejection. We cover this with increased topical steroids for at least 1 month, as well as antibiotics.

Toric Intraocular Lens

A very attractive option is the use of a toric intraocular lens (IOL), either alone or in combination with corneal surgery. Current astigmatic correction with IOLs is limited to 2 D at the corneal plane, but this limit is expected to increase. IOL-based toric correction is inherently geometrically symmetrical. However, if corneal surgery such as AK or laser vision correction can reduce the patient to moderate amounts of reasonably regular astigmatism, then the toric IOL can provide a highly accurate residual correction and result in excellent uncorrected and spectacle-corrected visual acuity.

References

1. Filatov V, Steinert RF, Talamo JH. Postkeratoplasty astigmatism with single running suture or interrupted sutures. *Am J Ophthalmol.* 1993;115(6):715-721.
2. Filatov V, Alexandrakis GF, Talamo JH, Steinert RF. Comparison of suture-in and suture-out postkeratoplasty astigmatism with single running suture or combined running and interrupted sutures. *Am J Ophthalmol.* 1996;122(5):696-700.

FINANCIAL DISCLOSURES

Dr. Natalie A. Afshari has no financial or proprietary interest in the materials presented herein. Dr. Afshari receives a research grant from National Eye Institute.

Dr. Anthony J. Aldave has no financial or proprietary interest in the materials presented herein.

Dr. Penny Asbell has no financial or proprietary interest in the materials presented herein.

Dr. Dimitri T. Azar has no financial or proprietary interest in the materials presented herein.

Dr. Neal P. Barney has no financial or proprietary interest in the materials presented herein.

Dr. Michael W. Belin has no financial or proprietary interest in the materials presented herein.

Dr. Richard E. Braunstein has no financial or proprietary interest in the materials presented herein.

Dr. Daniel Brocks has no financial or proprietary interest in the materials presented herein.

Dr. JoAnn C. Chang has no financial or proprietary interest in the materials presented herein.

Dr. David S. Chu is a speaker for Alcon, Allergan, Inspire, Sirion, and Vistakon, and he receives research support from Lux Bio and Novartis.

Dr. John W. Cowden discloses that the preparation of this chapter was supported in part by an unrestricted grant from Research to Prevent Blindness, New York, NY. Dr. Cowden has no financial interests in any pharmaceutical companies related to the medications mentioned in this chapter.

Dr. Reza Dana has no financial or proprietary interest in the materials presented herein.

Dr. Muriel Doors has no financial or proprietary interest in the materials presented herein.

Dr. James P. Dunn has no financial or proprietary interest in the materials presented herein.

Dr. Brad H. Feldman has no financial or proprietary interest in the materials presented herein.

Dr. Martin Filipec has no financial or proprietary interest in the materials presented herein.

Dr. C. Stephen Foster has no financial or proprietary interest in the materials presented herein.

Dr. Frederick (Rick) W. Fraunfelder has no financial or proprietary interest in the materials presented herein.

Dr. Prashant Garg is a consultant and member of the speaker's buraeu for Alcon International.

Dr. Kenneth Mark Goins has no financial or proprietary interest in the materials presented herein.

Dr. Mark S. Gorovoy has no financial or proprietary interest in the materials presented herein.

Dr. Jose L. Güell has no financial or proprietary interest in the materials presented herein.

Dr. Sadeer B. Hannush has no financial or proprietary interest in the materials presented herein.

Dr. Bennie H. Jeng has no financial or proprietary interest in the materials presented herein.

Dr. Albert S. Jun has no financial or proprietary interest in the materials presented herein.

Dr. Stephen C. Kaufman has no financial or proprietary interest in the materials presented herein.

Dr. Tanya Khan has no financial or proprietary interest in the materials presented herein.

Dr. Terry Kim has no financial or proprietary interest in the materials presented herein.

Dr. Thomas Kohnen has no financial or proprietary interest in the materials presented herein.

Dr. Aarup A. Kubal has no financial or proprietary interest in the materials presented herein.

Dr. Marian Macsai has no financial or proprietary interest in the materials presented herein.

Dr. Francis S. Mah has interest in Alcon, Allergan, Inspire, InSite, and Ista.

Dr. Mark J. Mannis has no financial or proprietary interest in the materials presented herein.

Dr. Thomas F. Mauger has no financial or proprietary interest in the materials presented herein.

Dr. Jod S. Mehta has no financial or proprietary interest in the materials presented herein.

Dr. Merce Morral has no financial or proprietary interest in the materials presented herein.

Dr. Majid Moshirfar has no financial or proprietary interest in the materials presented herein.

Dr. John D. Ng is a consultant and shareholder for Natures Tears Eye Mist, Bio-Logic Aqua, Inc.

Dr. Rudy M. M. A. Nuijts has no financial or proprietary interest in the materials presented herein.

Dr. Michael A. Page has not disclosed any relevant financial relationships.

Dr. Carlindo Da Reitz Pereira has no financial or proprietary interest in the materials presented herein.

Dr. Henry Daniel Perry is a consultant for Allergan and Inspire.

Dr. Stephen C. Pflugfelder has no financial or proprietary interest in the materials presented herein.

Dr. Roberto Pineda is a consultant for Alcon and part of the speaker's bureau for Allergan.

Dr. Yaron S. Rabinowitz is a consultant for Abbott Medical Optics.

Dr. Michael B. Raizman has no financial or proprietary interest in the materials presented herein.

Dr. J. Bradley Randleman has no financial or proprietary interest in the materials presented herein.

Dr. Virender S. Sangwan has no financial or proprietary interest in the materials presented herein.

Dr. Hosam Sheha has not disclosed any relevant financial relationships.

Dr. Mohamed Abou Shousha has no financial or proprietary interest in the materials presented herein.

Dr. Sana S. Siddique has no financial or proprietary interest in the materials presented herein.

Dr. Roger F. Steinert has no financial or proprietary interest in the materials presented herein.

Dr. Donald Tan has no financial or proprietary interest in the materials presented herein.

Dr. Joseph Tauber has no financial or proprietary interest in the materials presented herein.

Dr. Mark A. Terry has no financial or proprietary interest in the materials presented herein.

Dr. Kristina Thomas has no financial or proprietary interest in the materials presented herein.

Dr. Prathima R. Thumma has not disclosed any relevant financial relationships.

Dr. William Trattler is a consultant and received research funding/speaking honoraria for Allergan, Inspire, Ista, Abbott Medical Optics, Vistakon, Lenstec, Glaukos, Sirion Therapeutics, QLTI, Wavetec, and Bausch & Lomb.

Dr. Scheffer C. G. Tseng is a shareholder of TissueTech, Inc., which owns US patents 6,152,142 and 6,326,019 on the method of preparation and clinical uses of human amniotic membrane, and ProKera, distributed by Bio-Tissue Inc.

Dr. Elmer Y. Tu has no financial or proprietary interest in the materials presented herein.

Dr. David D. Verdier has no financial or proprietary interest in the materials presented herein.

Dr. Nienke Visser has no financial or proprietary interest in the materials presented herein.

Dr. Carroll A. Webers has no financial or proprietary interest in the materials presented herein.

Dr. Jayne S. Weiss is part of the speaker's bureau for Alcon.

Dr. Sonia H. Yoo has no financial or proprietary interest in the materials presented herein.

INDEX

Wait...There's More!

SLACK Incorporated's Health Care Books and Journals offers a wide selection of books in the field of Ophthalmology. We are dedicated to providing important works that educate, inform and improve the knowledge of our customers. Don't miss out on our other informative titles that will enhance your collection.

The exciting and unique *Curbside Consultation Series* is designed to effectively provide ophthalmologists with practical, to the point, evidence based answers to the questions most frequently asked during informal consultations between colleagues.

Each specialized book included in the *Curbside Consultation Series* offers quick access to current medical information with the ease and convenience of a conversation. Expert consultants who are recognized leaders in their fields provide their advice, preferences, and opinions to answer the tricky questions that require ophthalmologists to practice the "art" of medicine.

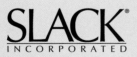